Emergency Cross-cover of Surgical Specialties

Emergency Cross-cover of Surgical Specialties:

A Survival Guide

Edited by

Robert Miller

Cambridge
Scholars
Publishing

Emergency Cross-cover of Surgical Specialties: A Survival Guide

Edited by Robert Miller

This book first published 2020

Cambridge Scholars Publishing

Lady Stephenson Library, Newcastle upon Tyne, NE6 2PA, UK

British Library Cataloguing in Publication Data
A catalogue record for this book is available from the British Library

ISBN (10): 1-5275-4334-X
ISBN (13): 978-1-5275-4334-8

TABLE OF CONTENTS

List of Figures and Illustrations ... vii

List of Tables ... xii

Foreword ... xiv

Preface ... xv

Acknowledgements ... xvi

Introduction ... xvii
Robert Miller

List of Abbreviations ... xxii

Chapter 1 ... 1
Breast Surgery
Virginia Caddick & Abdul Kasem

Chapter 2 ... 17
Ear, Nose and Throat Surgery
Jessica Lunn & Raj Lakhani

Chapter 3 ... 56
General Surgery
Simon McCluney & Christos Kontovounisios

Chapter 4 ... 84
Oral and Maxillofacial Surgery
Zachary Cole-Healy, Toby Visholm & Indran Balasundaram

Chapter 5 ... 108
Paediatric Surgery
Simon McCluney & Iain Yardley

Chapter 6 127
Plastic Surgery
Mark Mikhail & Sally Jay

Chapter 7 154
Trauma and Orthopaedics
Oliver Beaumont & Oliver Gosling.

Chapter 8 182
Urology
John Pascoe & Jennifer Martin

Chapter 9 234
Vascular Surgery
Tom Pampiglione

Chapter 10 255
Medical Emergencies in Surgery
Sam McGrath & Kevin O'Gallagher

Chapter 11 292
Helpful Websites and Mobile Applications
Hugo Beaumont & Robert Miller

Editor Biography 298

List of Contributors 299

List of Figures and Illustrations

Chapter 1: Breast Surgery

- Figure 1. *Diagram of documenting in clock-face and quadrants*
- Figure 2. *Wide local excision*
- Figure 3. *Mastectomy*
- Figure 4. *Sentinel lymph node biopsy*
- Figure 5. *Axillary lymph node biopsy*
- Figure 6. *Therapeutic mammoplasty*
- Figure 7. *Breast reduction (symmetrising)*
- Figure 8. *Mastopexy (symmetrising)*
- Figure 9. *Implant based reconstruction +/- acellular dermal matrix*
- Figure 10. *Latissimus dorsi*
- Figure 11. *Deep inferior epigastric artery reconstruction*

Chapter 2: Ear, Nose and Throat

- Figure 1. *The ENT bag*
- Figure 2. *Flexible Nasendoscopy*
- Figure 3. *Weber and Rinne Tests. A) The Weber Test B) The Rinne Test: Tines in front of the ear C) The Rinne Test: Footplate on the mastoid*
- Figure 4. *Anterior rhinoscopy: A) Holding nasal thudichums; B) Anterior rhinoscopy*
- Figure 5. *Differential diagnosis of facial nerve palsy*
- Figure 6. *Top tips for SSNHL*
- Figure 7. *Acquired Causes of sensorineural hearing loss*
- Figure 8. *Red flags for malignant otitis externa*
- Figure 9. *Otitis Externa Top Tips*
- Figure 10. *A) crocodile forceps B) pope wick C) pope wick insertion*
- Figure 11. *Topical treatment for otitis externa*
- Figure 12. *Aural Foreign bodies Top Tips*
- Figure 13. *Complication of Otitis Media*
- Figure 14. *A) Normal ear anatomy B) Pinna block*
- Figure 15. *Incision of pinna haematoma*

- Figure 16. *Drainage of pinna haematoma and compression using sialastic splints following drainage of pinna haematoma*
- Figure 17. *Risk Factors/ Underlying Aetiology of Epistaxis*
- Figure 18. *Epistaxis management top tips*
- Figure 19. *Anterior Nasal Packing. Illustration and step wise approach*
- Figure 20. *Septal haematoma*
- Figure 21. *Nasal Foreign Bodies*
- Figure 22. *Jobson Horne Probe*
- Figure 23. *Sore Throat differential diagnosis*
- Figure 24. *Criteria for Tonsillectomy* (The Scottish Intercollegiate Guidelines Network)
- Figure 25. *A) Normal oropharynx B) Tonsillitis C) Peritonsillar abscess*
- Figure 26. *Peritonsillar abscess drainage*
- Figure 27. *Differential Diagnosis of Acute Stridor*
- Figure 28. *Initial Management of Stridor*

Chapter 3: General Surgery

- Figure 1. *A) Abdominal radiograph demonstrating small bowel obstruction; B) Axial image of a computerised tomography scan demonstrating small bowel obstruction. The red arrow indicates the air/fluid level typical of bowel obstruction*
- Figure 2. *Abdominal radiograph demonstrating sigmoid volvulus with the characteristic coffee bean sign*
- Figure 3. *Coronal and axial slices of a computerised tomography scan demonstrating a large pancreatic pseudocyst with compression with the left renal vessels*
- Figure 4. *A) A schematic demonstrating inguinal herniae anatomy; B) An axial slice of a computerised tomography scan of an incarcerated left inguinal hernia containing bowel*
- Figure 5. *Internal and external haemorrhoids*
- Figure 6. *Types of perianal fistulae based on their location in relation to the anal sphincters*
- Figure 7. *Images demonstrating: A) Roux-en-Y gastric bypass; B) B) adjustable gastric band*
- Figure 8. *Erect chest radiograph demonstrating free intra-peritoneal air under the right hemi-diaphragm*

Chapter 4: Oral and Maxillofacial Surgery

- Figure 1. *Simplified training pathway for OMFS*
- Figure 2. *Simplified tooth anatomy*
- Figure 3. *Set square diagram. Imagine as if you are looking at the patients mouth from the front*

Chapter 5: Paediatric Surgery

- Figure 1. *Diagram illustrating the process of intussusception*
- Figure 2. Ultrasound demonstrating the classical target sign in intussusception
- Figure 3. *Intestinal pneumatosis in a child with NEC*

Chapter 6: Plastic Surgery

- Figure 1. *Hand and forearm – dermatomes*
- Figure 2. *Major forearm nerves and arteries*
- Figure 3. *Examining for FDP and FDS anatomy and examination*
- Figure 4. *Assessment of burn depth – Taken from the LSEBN Burn Depth Assessment Guidance* (LSEBN 2015a)
- Figure 5. *Ring block technique*
- Figure 6. *Lund and Browder diagram for adults – The percentage values for the head, upper and lower legs are then adjusted for depending on the age of the child* (*Adapted from Grabb and Smith: Plastic Surgery* [Klein 2007*]).*
- Figure 7. *HIPE app interface with example of pathway for hand laceration injuries (left to right). Selected options highlighted in red.*

Chapter 7: Trauma and Orthopaedics

- Figure 1. *The Lethal Triad observed in trauma scenarios*
- Figure 2. *Locations for 3-point fixation in a wrist fracture. Note how the intact periosteal hinge acts to align the fracture*
- Figure 3. *Gilulas arcs in blue on an AP radiograph of the wrist. The red arrow points to a scaphoid waist fracture*
- Figure 4. *Demonstrates appearances on AP shoulder radiographs. A) Anterior shoulder dislocation; B) Posterior shoulder dislocation; C) Hill-Sachs and Bankart lesions post reduction of a different shoulder.*
- Figure 5. *Neck of femur fracture classification: 'subcapital (intracapsular)', intertrochanteric (extracapsular) and subtrochanteric (extracapsular)*

- Figure 6. *Ankle fracture patterns and associated ligamentous injuries*
- Figure 7. *AP Radiography of a bimalleolar right ankle fracture. blue arrow=Talar shift, orange = increased medial clear space, green=tib/fib overlap, measured 1cm above the joint line (<5mm is abnormal on mortise view XR)*
- Figure 8. *AP Radiograph of the left foot showing a LisFranc Injury with increased gap and evidence of a bony fracture fragment between the 1st and 2nd ray*
- Figure 9. *Diagrammatic section of a sagittal section through the lumbar spine illustrating the position of the three spinal columns*
- Figure 10. *Lateral XR of the Cervical spine, with each vertebrae numbered and lines to demonstrate: anterior vertebral line (blue), posterior vertebral line (yellow), spino-laminar line (red), posterior spinous line (green)*
- Figure 11. *Diagram illustrating the Salter Harris classification for fractures involving the epiphysis of long bones*
- Figure 12. *Radiograph of paediatric left hip. Klein's line drawn along superior aspect of femoral neck – A slipped upper femoral epiphysis is evident as the line does not intersect the femoral head.*
- Figure 13. *a) Lateral radiograph of an uninjured skeletally immature elbow. Red = radiocapitellar line, blue = anterior humeral line b) Lateral radiograph of a skeletally mature elbow, demonstrating anterior and posterior fat pad signs*

Chapter 8: Urology

- Figure 1. *Testicular pain*
- Figure 2. *An animal demonstration comparing testicular torsion. Normal, Left & Torted, Right*
- Figure 3. *Management pathways for testicular torsion*
- Figure 4. *X-Ray KUB of a large left renal stone and distal stones*
- Figure 5. *Illustration of nephrostomy placement.*
- Figure 6. *An XRay KUB with a right JJ ureteric stent in situ.*
- Figure 7. *A visibly distended bladder – a rare sign that may be seen in urinary retention.*
- Figure 8. *Flank Pain*
- Figure 9. *Rectal Exam – note the position of the prostate.*
- Figure 10. *Ultrasound showing evidence of hydronephrosis.*
- Figure 11. *Curved tip catheter.*
- Figure 12. *Public patient information notice on urine colour.*

- Figure 13. *Three-way catheter*
- Figure 14. *Paraphimosis and phimosis*
- Figure 15. *Cross-section of the penis. When aspirating a priapism, the needle should enter at the 2 & 10 o'clock position avoiding the vasculature & urethra.*
- Figure 16. *A patient after extensive debridement for Fournier's gangrene. Note the urethral catheter in situ and colostomy bag.*

Chapter 9: Vascular Surgery - N/A

Chapter 10: Medical Emergencies in Surgery
- Figure 1. *Top tips for ECG interpretation*
- Figure 2. *SOCRATES pain mnemonic*
- Figure 3. *Post-operative atelectasis*
- Figure 4. *Reversible risk factors for AF*
- Figure 5: *ECG showing atrial fibrillation. There is no evidence of p-waves, the rhythm is irregular (the distance between each QRS complex is different).*
- Figure 6. *Cardiac risk factors*
- Figure 7. *Differential diagnoses for chest pain*
- Figure 9. *STEMI criteria*
- Figure 10. *Pulmonary embolism risk factors*
- Figure 11. *Wells criteria for Pulmonary Embolism*
- Figure 12. Signs for immediate escalation
- Figure 13. *ECG changes in hyperkalaemia*
- Figure 14. *ECG showing tall tented t waves in v3 –v6, leads II & III classical of hyperkalaemia*
- Figure 15. *Diagnostic criteria for DKA*
- Figure 16. *Factors require immediate escalation for HDU in DKA*
- Figure 17. *The importance of potassium in DKA*
- Figure 18. *Diagnosis of HHS*

Chapter 11: Helpful Websites and Mobile Applications - N/A

LIST OF TABLES

Chapter 1: Breast Surgery
- N/A

Chapter 2: Ear, Nose and Throat
- Table 1. *Interpretation of Rinne and Weber tests*
- Table 2. *Idiopathic facial nerve palsy versus other pathology*

Chapter 3: General Surgery
- Table 1. *The Alvarado Score*
- Table 2. *Glasgow Acute Pancreatitis Severity Score*

Chapter 4: Oral and Maxillofacial Surgery
- N/A

Chapter 5: Paediatric Surgery
- N/A

Chapter 6: Plastic Surgery
- Table 1. *Flap observations*
- Table 2. *Gustillo-Anderson Classification of open tib/fib fractures*
- Table 3. *LRINEC scoring*

Chapter 7: Trauma and Orthopaedics
- Table 1. *The Gustilo and Anderson Classification of Open Fractures (Gustilo and Anderson, 1976)*
- Table 2. *Details the normal parameters for anatomy of the distal radius and what change to accept in a displaced fracture.*

Chapter 8: Urology
- Table 1. *Differential diagnosis for testicular torsion*
- Table 2. *Differential diagnosis for ureteric colic*
- Table 3. *American Association for the Surgery of Trauma grading for renal trauma*

Chapter 9: Vascular Surgery
- Table 1. *Pain questions*
- Table 2. *Pulse Anatomy*
- Table 3. *ABPI interpretation*

Chapter 10: Medical Emergencies in Surgery
- N/A

Chapter 11: Helpful Websites and Mobile Applications
- N/A

FOREWORD

PROFESSOR SIMON MYERS

In austere times, staff efficiencies in the NHS are often criticised. In a more positive approach, Robert Miller has been realistic and pragmatic about cross-cover arrangements, and very helpfully, alongside others with experience at SHO grade, provided support for those managing patients outside their primary specialty interest. The content is inevitably selective, and could never be exhaustive. It comes across, however, as well conceived, and illustrated. It will fill the gaps whilst SHOs find their feet in a post, and is likely to be embraced by other team members e.g. clinical nurse specialists. It will encourage informed discussion with senior grades. The authors should be congratulated for sharing their experiences in the interests of others challenged in the same way, and in the interests of patient care. It should become a staple for relevant departmental induction programmes.

Professor Simon Myers PhD FRCS [Plast]

GAPS Professor of Academic Plastic Surgery [Queen Mary University] & Honorary Consultant Plastic, Burn, Reconstructive & Aesthetic Surgeon [Barts & The London NHS Healthcare Trust]

PREFACE

This book has been designed to support the performance of junior doctors working at senior house officer level across surgical subspecialties. The hope is that it will improve both the standard of care given to patients and the efficiency and experience of doctors providing such care during on-call duties.

ACKNOWLEDGEMENTS

Illustrations:

The illustrations seen throughout this book have been designed and produced by **Ginny Caddick**. Ginny is a London-based General Surgery trainee working as a Registrar in the South East London Deanery. With clinical experience in General and Plastic Surgery, she hopes to pursue a career in Oncoplastic Breast Surgery. However, in her spare time, she has developed a keen interest in an assortment of artistic modalities. These include etching, screen-printing and, as you can see, illustrating. She has been involved in a number of educational illustration projects, within biological science and medical fields. It has been a privilege to work with her in the production of the fantastic illustrations seen throughout this book.

Instagram: @thechirographer

Front cover:

The front cover has been designed by the very talented **Hugo Beaumont**. Hugo is currently working as a senior house officer in Bristol, but has a keen interest in art and graphic design. He has been involved in a number of medically-orientated projects including work as the graphic designer for the U.K. Sepsis Trust during the formative stages of the charity.

INTRODUCTION

ROBERT MILLER

With the introduction of the European Working Time Directive and changes to doctors' contracts and rotas, junior doctors at senior house officer (SHO) level are increasingly expected to cross-cover surgical specialties whilst on-call. Often these are specialties in which they have limited, or no, post-graduate experience or training. Departmental inductions are often short, rushed or missed altogether, particularly for those who only work in the specialty when providing cross-cover whilst on-call. It is not uncommon for SHOs to find themselves covering a speciality on-call for the first time out-of-hours, when senior supervision is less readily available. This can lead to inefficient delivery of patient care and be stressful. Many questions or situations faced whilst on-call are not life or limb threatening, but if the individual has little experience within the speciality, they simply find themselves unequipped with the day-to-day working knowledge to adequately provide answers or solutions. Whilst the answers may be found within textbooks or online, this is often not feasible during a busy on-call period and can lead to stress, anxiety and delays in patient care.

This book is **written for junior doctors, by junior doctors**. It aims to provide a **concise and easy to read tool** for doctors covering surgical specialties whilst on-call and is written by authors who have extensive experience in each speciality at SHO level. It covers each surgical speciality in turn, addressing speciality specific emergencies; when to admit patients; when to call for senior help and guidance on common referrals or questions post-operative complications and common medical emergencies in surgical patients. In addition, it outlines some key practical skills often required in surgical specialties, providing tips and tricks for performing them safely and successfully. Lastly, with increasing availability of high-quality Apps and websites, it summarises key online resources available for junior doctors within surgical specialties.

This book is the ideal companion for any junior doctor, physicians' assistants, emergency nurse practitioners or advance nurse practitioners involved in delivering care to surgical patients. The aim is to allow doctors to deliver high-quality patient care with confidence. The book does not aim to replace already available, high quality, anatomy resources. Much of surgery relies on a sound knowledge of relevant anatomy and this should be revised. Although this book aims to cover all the common situations and scenarios faced when on-call, if you are in doubt it is always acceptable and appropriate to contact your senior to ask for help, confirm your management plan or escalate an unwell patient.

What to establish prior to starting any on-call shift:

Before starting an on-call SHO shift in any surgical speciality, whether in or out-of-hours, there are some basic points you must familiarise yourself with in order to facilitate organised, efficient and safe delivery of care.

Below is a list of points that should be established prior to starting your shift. If you are working in an unfamiliar hospital or department, or as a locum doctor, it is completely reasonable for you to request these details prior to starting your shift.

- Your seniors:
    - Consultant on-call
    - Registrar on-call and contact details

- Referrals:
    - What external units do you accept referrals from
    - What cases do you accept/not accept

- Helpful contact numbers:
    - On-call medical team
    - Intensive care team and outreach team
    - Site/bed manager
    - On-call radiologist and on-call radiographer/mobile imaging

- Documentation and computer systems:
    - Computer log-in details
    - Where to document patient reviews on the ward and in A&E
    - Speciality specific computer system and log-in details

    - How to access the in-patient and clinic lists
    - Imaging system and log-in details

- Booking theatre cases:
    - Theatre case booking – online, hand-written or both?
    - On-call anaesthetist contact details
    - Theatre co-ordinator contact details

- Bloods:
    - How to request (hand written or printed)
    - How to send (porter or pod system)
    - Group and save process (online, hand written, printed and how many samples)

- Hot and cold clinics:
    - How to book into them
    - What to tell the patient
    - What cases can or should be booked and suitable timeframes

- Abscess pathways:
    - Almost all surgical specialties will have an abscess pathway for cases that require operative management but do not require admission.
    - How to book into them and what to tell the patient

- Local microbiology guidelines

The below points should be established when receiving a hand-over at the beginning of your shift to ensure the safe continuity of care.

- Patients awaiting review in A&E or awaiting senior review

- Unwell patients:
    - Patients to be aware of
    - Patients to review
    - Escalation plans for these patients from the day team if covering nights

- Post-operative patients:
    - Post-operative patients that require review overnight

- Post-operative patients to be aware of
- Post-operative bloods to review, chase, or request

- Pre-operative patients:
    - Elective or emergency cases that have been admitted for surgery
    - Overnight it is important to ensure these patients have been appropriately worked-up for theatre (bloods, ECG, X-ray etc…)
    - Remember to add them to the patient list

Preparing patients for theatre

As a surgical SHO it is vital that you are able to ensure patients that require surgery are appropriately worked up and ready for surgery so there are no delays.

Delays caused by poor preparation or planning are almost always preventable and cause much frustration to theatre teams and delay patients' care.

Compulsory items:

- Signed consent form for the procedure:
    - If you are not familiar with the procedure and the possible risks and complications, ask for senior help or inform your team that you have not been able to consent the patient
    - Including surgical site
    - Remember to include any additional procedures that may be performed such as placing nasogastric tube, catheters and drains
    - If the patient cannot consent, a consent Form 4 should be completed by a senior member of the team with family/next of kin involvement

- Mark the surgical site and confirm this with the patient (if possible)
- Book the patient for theatre/ensure they are on the operating list (theatre co-ordinator and anaesthetic team need to be aware but the exact process depends on your hospital).

- Ensure nil by mouth status clarified and both the patient and nursing staff are aware:
    - 6 hours pre-operatively for food and most drinks
    - 2 hours pre-operatively for clear fluids (water, black coffee, black tea, non-fizzy diluted juice)
    - Although this is the traditional guidance and is often adopted, there is evidence to suggest that these criteria are too strict and hence there is inter-hospital variation

Procedure dependent items:

- Blood group and screen. Ensure the correct number of bottles have been sent/ labelled correctly. Check with the blood bank for high risk patients
- Cross match units of blood if applicable
- Coagulation studies
- FBC & U&Es
- ECG (patients >50 years, or if clinically indicated)
- CXR (patients >50 years, or if clinically indicated, undergoing GA or abdominal surgery)
- Foley catheter to monitor fluid status (if applicable)
- Anaesthetic consultation/review pre-op
- Reserved monitored bed post-operatively (if applicable)
    - Patient undergoing complex free flap reconstruction and head and neck cases need to be managed on wards competent in monitoring free flaps or complex airways
- Procedure specific imaging

Addressing the points raised throughout this section will ensure you are effective whilst working on-call. This will in turn facilitate the delivery of excellent patient care. However, despite all efforts, on-call working can be tough and stressful (we have all had a shift that haunts us!). Remember, always take a break and have something to eat /drink and if you are struggling, ask for support.

LIST OF ABBREVIATIONS

AAA	Abdominal Aortic Aneurysm
AAST	American Association for the Surgeons of Trauma
ABPI	Ankle Brachial Pressure Index
ACS	Acute Coronary Syndrome
AF	Atrial Fibrillation
ALI	Acute Limb Ischaemia
AMTS	Abbreviated Mental Test Score
AP	Anterior-Posterior
ATLS	Advanced Trauma Life Support
AVPU	Alert, Voice, Pain, Unresponsive
BAUS	British Association of Urologists
BOAST	British Orthopaedic Association Standards for Trauma
BPH	Benign Prostatic Hyperplasia
CI	Intermittent Claudication
CLI	Critical Limb Ischaemia
CLI	Critical Limb Ischaemia
COPD	Chronic Obstructive Pulmonary Disease
CRP	C-reactive protein
CT	Computed Tomography
CXR	Chest X-Ray
DJ	Duodeno-jejunal
DKA	Diabetic Ketoacidosis
DPT	Dental Panoramic Tomography
DRE	Digital Rectal Examination
DRUJ	distal radio-ulnar joint
EAU	European association of Urology
ECG	Electrocardiogram
ED	Emergency Department
EMSB	Emergency Management of Severe Burns
ENT	Ear Nose and Throat
FBC	Full Blood Count
GA	General Anaesthetic
G&S	Group and Save
GCS	Glasgow Coma Scale
GP	General Practitioner
HAP	Hospital Acquired Pneumonia

HHS	Hyperosmolar Hyperglycaemic Syndrome
IV	Intra-venous
KUB	Kidney, Urethral, Bladder
LUTS	Lower Urinary Tract Symptoms
LA	Local Anaesthetic
MC&S	Microscopy, culture and sensitivities
MRI	Magnetic Resonance Imaging
MTC	Major Trauma Centre
MUA	Manipulation under anaesthetic
NBM	Nil by Mouth
NGT	Nasogastric tube
NICE	National Institute of Clinical Excellence
NSAID	Non-Steroidal Anti-Inflammatory Drug
OM	Occipitomental
OMFS	Oral and Maxillofacial Surgery
ORIF	Open reduction internal fixation
PA	Posterior to Anterior
PCI	Percutaneous Coronary Intervention
PCN	Percutaneous nephrostomy
PSA	Prostate Specific Antigen
SHO	Senior House Officer
SPC	Supra-pubic catheter
SSNHL	Sudden onset SensoriNeural Hearing Loss
STI	Sexually transmitted infection
T&O	Trauma and Orthopaedics
TBSA	Total Body Surface Area
TWOC	Trial Without Catheter
U&E	Urea and Electrolytes
USS	Ultrasound scan
UTI	Urinary Tract Infection
WBC	White Blood Cells

CHAPTER 1

BREAST SURGERY

VIRGINIA CADDICK & ABDUL KASEM

Abstract
Section 1 – Introduction
Section 2 – Breast History
Section 3 – Breast Examination
Section 4 – Common Presenting Complaints
  Breast abscess
  Axillary abscess
  Fungating breast lesions
  Breast Haematomas
  Seroma
  Implant problems
  Nipple necrosis
Section 5 – Review of Inpatients
  Wide local excision
  Mastectomy
  Sentinel lymph node biopsy
  Axillary node clearance
  Therapeutic mammoplasty
  Breast reduction (symmetrising)
  Mastopexy (symmetrising)
  Implant based reconstruction +/- Acellular dermal matrix
Section 6 – Autologous breast reconstruction
  Latissimus dorsi
  Deep inferior epigastric artery
Section 7 – How to manage a free flap

Abstract

Breast surgery is often encompassed within general surgery but can be a stand-alone surgical speciality and comes with specific considerations when on-call.

This chapter covers key breast pathologies and treatment principles encountered when providing cross-cover care. It will also cover general principles regarding understanding and managing elective breast patients on the ward.

Section 1: Introduction

As a surgical Foundation Year 2 doctor or core trainee on-call, you will encounter a variety of breast patients. This chapter endeavours to prepare you to deal with the most common presentations. These fall in to 2 main categories:

- New presentations (as GP or ED referrals)
- Post-operative complications:
    - In-patient ward reviews
    - Re-admissions:
        - Locally NHS treated patients
        - Private sector cosmetic patients

First, we will explore a standardised approach to history taking and examination when clerking or reviewing breast patients.

Section 2: History Taking in Breast Patients:

Presenting complaints:

- Is there a lump?
- Is there any breast pain? Cyclical/non-cyclical; unilateral/bilateral
- Are there any skin changes?
- Nipple discharge: Uniductal/multiductal/spontaneous. Colour: blood-stained, milky/clear, green/brown
- Nipple changes: inversion

To assess risk of breast cancer:

- Age of menarche
- Age of menopause
- Years of OCP/HRT
- Number of children (and number breast fed)
- Previous breast cancer:
    - Laterality, date of diagnosis
    - Histology
    - Surgery
    - Adjuvant treatment
- BMI
- Smoking
- Family history

Implants:

- Uni/bilateral
- Date of previous procedures, consultant
- Implant type:
    - Expander or implant
    - Size
    - Shape/brand
- Any previous implant problems:
    - History of wound problems
    - History of infection

Section 3: Breast Examination

All patients, especially in acute presentations or post-operative patients, should be examined within the context of an ABCDE framework. Breast examination would take place in 'Exposure'. It is important to review the observations, the medication chart, the pain chart and any operative/ward notes.

A: AIRWAY
B: BREATHING
C: CIRCULATION
D: DISABILITY
E: EXPOSURE

Patient Positioning: Ideally Patients should be examined both at 45 degrees, with arm above head, and sat on edge of bed with hands on hips. All patients should be examined without bra, and with chaperone.

Approach all 4 quadrants in a logical, systemised approach:

- Radial
- Spiral
- Quadrants
- Lumps:
    - Location in relation to quadrant/clock face
    - Size
    - Consistency - Is it fluctuant or firm?
    - Is it fixed or mobile? Is it tethered?
    - Is it tender?

Figure 1. *Diagram of documenting in clock-face and quadrants*
See colour centrefold for this image.

Are there overlying skin changes?

- Axilla:
    - Is there lymphadenopathy?
    - Is there a collection?
    - Is there an abscess?

- Nipple areolar complex:
    - Is it viable?
    - Are there any underlying collections?
- Post-operative patients with wounds/dressings:
    - Are the dressings dry/intact?
    - Is there an area of swelling/exquisite tenderness above that expected post-operatively?
- Drains:
    - What volume in i) last hour; and ii) last 24 hours
    - Contents: serosanguinous, serous, frank blood
    - Surrounding skin: any evidence of infection/ moisture lesions? Is the drain bypassing?

How to document breast lumps can be seen in figure 1. Accurate documentation is vital.

Section 4: Common Presenting Complaints

Depending on your local trust referral pathway, the majority of these patients can be seen in Breast Clinic. We will cover the most common presenting complaints that may be referred during an on call. These fall into 2 main categories:

New presentations:

1. Breast Abscess
2. Axillary abscesses
3. Fungating breast lesions
4. Breast trauma/haematomas

Post-operative complications:

1. Haematoma
2. Seroma/infected seroma
3. Implant problems

Breast abscess:

A suspected breast abscess is a common acute presentation to the General Surgery on call take. If there are clinical concerns regarding the following, they should be seen on the acute take rather than direct urgent breast clinic referral:

- Evidence of sepsis/systemic infection
- Evidence of skin necrosis warranting I&D on CEPOD
- Immunocompromise: e.g. diabetes

It most commonly affects women between the ages from 18-50. Aetiology can be divided into 2 groups: lactational and non-lactational abscesses. It is important to differentiate between mastitis and an abscess; the management for each is different.

In the History, ask about:

- Duration of symptoms
- Can they feel a lump? Has the size of this changed?
- Has it given out any pus?
- Have they had previous abscesses?

- Have they had previous skin infections (e.g. hidradenitis) or TB?
- Have they felt feverish/shivery?
- Are there any co-morbidities compromising immune system?
    - Diabetes Mellitus
    - Steroids
    - Immunosuppressants
    - BBV
- Do they smoke?
- Are they post-partum? If so, are they breastfeeding?
- Have they taken any antibiotics?
    - Which ones and duration of each course
    - Have they had any swabs taken? If so, where?

On Examination:

- Observations: Evidence of sepsis
    - Pyrexial
    - Tachycardia
    - SIRS response
- Breast:
    - Site of the lump (clock-face or quadrant)
    - Size
    - Fluctuance
    - Quality/involvement of overlying skin (necrosis/cellulitis)
    - Is there a discharging sinus/pus?

- Axilla: Is there palpable axillary lymphadenopathy?

Investigations:

- Bloods: inflammatory markers (WCC, neutrophil count, CRP)
- VBG if septic
- Cultures: blood, urine, pus swab
- Ultrasound +/- aspirate: is there a drainable collection? If so, specify need to send aspirate for microbiology!

Management:

Although like other abscesses, breast abscesses involve a walled-off collection of pus, often not adequately penetrated by oral antibiotics, the approach to drainage is different. A large cutaneous incision and healing by secondary intent is not usually appropriate in such a cosmetically important area.

1) Management of Sepsis:
    a) If evidence of sepsis, utilise ABCDE approach and apply 'septic 6' management principle (using appropriate trust guidance).
    b) If septic, admission for IV antibiotics, IVI and urgent drainage of abscess (ideally US-guided).
2) Referral to Breast Clinic:
    a) Most trusts have a breast abscess pathway. These patients are best managed in a breast clinic by experienced clinicians and breast radiologists.
    b) If high index of suspicion for breast abscess and discharging patient out of hours with referral to breast clinic, it is important to ensure patient is covered with oral antibiotics prior to review.
    c) Many abscesses are adequately drained radiologically, avoiding unnecessary scars from I&Ds in a cosmetically important area. This is compounded by the fact breast abscesses are recurrent. Countless I&Ds would lead to a poor aesthetic outcome.
3) Consideration of the Microbiology:
    a) Lactational versus non-lactational
    b) Review of pus MCS
    c) Following local trust antimicrobial guidance
    d) Consideration of patient's allergies/ contraindications in pregnancy/breast-feeding
    e) Discussion with Consultant microbiologist if complex case or atypical infections suspected

Axillary abscesses

- These do need to be seen on the acute General Surgery take and managed using the standard abscess pathway. They often require incision and drainage on the CEPOD list (if large enough/fluctuant/jeopardising overlying skin).
- They do not usually need to be seen by Breast team

Fungating breast lesions

Patients may be referred to surgical team via inpatient referral, GP or ED with fungating breast lesions.

These patients must be seen by a Breast team directly, ideally in a One Stop Clinic environment. This clinical setting enables appropriate work up (i.e. triple assessment and MDT discussion).

However, if the referring clinician is insistent on your review, you should discuss with your senior or local breast team.

Breast haematomas

Breast haematomas are most commonly either post-operative complications or the result of breast trauma.

History Taking & Examination - Breast Trauma:

- Mechanism of injury
- Site and extent
- Are there any other injuries?
- Are the pattern of injuries compatible with the history?
- Safeguarding concerns
- Consent for medical photography
- Medication history/ history of bleeding disorders/coagulopathy

It is important to consider that breast haematomas (like abscesses) can be atypical presentations of locally advanced breast cancers. For this reason, it is crucial that they too are managed directly by the breast team, with triple assessment and MDT discussion.

Breast haematomas need to be seen acutely on General Surgery take if:

a) There is a concern over active bleeding/expansile haematoma
b) Post-operative complications
c) Symptom control (i.e patient discomfort)
d) Overlying skin is not viable
e) Coagulopathy

Management:

Patients will require:

1) Bloods and intravenous access: Hb, clotting, group & save
2) Monitoring for evidence of haemodynamic instability
3) Marking of haematoma
4) Imaging if available

5) Urgent senior review if evidence of expanding haematoma or haemodynamic instability
6) Prep for theatre
7) Medication review (especially antiplatelets and anticoagulants)

Seroma

Seromas are a collection of serous fluid in the subcutaneous tissues. They are a common post-operative complication, particularly following mastectomy and axillary node clearance.

Smaller ones can be managed directly by breast care nurses in the community or in Breast clinic. However, large or symptomatic ones may need to be seen on the acute take.

- If there is a palpable collection that is fluctuant but tense, they can be drained with a large bore cannula Escalate to a senior if you are not confident in performing this procedure. If the fluid is clear, this can be aspirated and discarded
- If the aspirate is cloudy/malodourous/purulent or if there is overlying cellulitis or pyrexia, aspirate must be sent for MCS (as part of sepsis 6).
- If there is concern over potential infected seroma, the patient may need to be admitted for IV antibiotics and potential washout in theatre.
- Is there an implant? Seromas associated with implants increase the risk of implant infection/loss. It is absolutely crucial if aspirating a seroma with an implant to consider the following:
    - Ensure sterile conditions as important not to introduce infection/contaminate implant cavity.
    - Ideally such procedures should be done under image (US) guidance, to avoid implant damage/rupture.

Implant problems

There are a number of implant problems that may be referred to either Breast or Plastics teams depending on the patient and their past surgical history. These include:

- Exposed implants
- Infected implants
- Concern regarding rupture

- Capsular contracture
- Contour defects/rippling

Usually, if there is a concern regarding exposure of an implant or infection, these patients must be seen acutely. Rupture, capsular contracture or contour defects can all be seen in the out-patient clinic setting.

Exposed implants/ infected implants:

A silicon implant is a foreign body. Contamination with microorganisms (i.e. if implant is exposed or infected) is therefore almost impossible to eradicate due to the formation of a bio-film. Therefore, in both cases, it is highly likely the implant will need to be removed in the acute setting.

In the history:

- Duration of symptoms
- Previous surgical history
- Any systemic symptoms?

Examination:

- Is there any wound dehiscence? If so, can you see any silicon implant (colourless, usually textured material within the wound).

Management:

- Admit
- Commence on IV antibiotics
- Ensure NBM
- Inform senior
- If comfortable, consent for exploration of wound +/- removal of implant and washout

Wound problems (dehiscence, delayed healing):

If there are wound problems, these often need to be urgently clinically assessed to ensure:

- There is no evidence of exposed implant
- No evidence of infection

- Swabs for microbiology
- Ensure appropriate dressings management

Implant rupture

These patients can often be seen in the out-patient setting (urgent appointment). Rupture is an indication for removal of implant/exchange. However, depending on the referral, there may be specific grounds for admission. If unsure, it is important to discuss with your senior.

Nipple necrosis

This is most likely to be an immediate post-operative concern. It most commonly occurs in procedures where the nipple has been mobilised or underlying duct procedures have been carried out. Occasionally it can be due to suturing and excess tissue tension or constricting dressings. It should therefore be urgently reviewed by senior. If however, necrosis has already occurred, it must be allowed to delineate and debridement planned. Nipple reconstruction is a common oncoplastic procedure with numerous techniques available and can be planned electively.

Section 5: Review of Inpatients

The majority of breast patients undergo procedures in the day case setting. However, some procedures, co-morbidities or complications warrant hospital admission. In order to adequately assess and manage these patients, it is crucial to understand the common procedures:

1. Wide Local Excision
2. Mastectomy
3. Sentinel Lymph Node Biopsy
4. Axillary Clearance
5. Therapeutic mammoplasty
6. (Symmetrising) breast reduction
7. (Symmetrising) mastopexy
8. Implant based reconstruction +/- Acellular Dermal Matrix (ADM)
9. Autologous breast reconstruction:
    a. Latissimus dorsi
    b. DIEP

Wide Local Excision

Figure 2. *Wide local excision*
See colour centrefold for this image.

Wide local excision is a common breast-conserving procedure to achieve oncological clearance. The tumour is excised with a margin of tissue around it.

Tumours are often localised radiologically with a wire: 'wire-guided wide local excision'.

Mastectomy

Entire breast excised as an oncological procedure.

Appropriate for:

- Locally advanced/large tumours
- Multifocal tumours
- Small breasted-patients in which breast conserving surgery would leave an anaesthetically poor outcome.

Figure 3. *Mastectomy*
See colour centrefold for this image.

Mastectomy can be divided into the following:

1) Mastectomy without immediate breast reconstruction:

a) **Simple mastectomy:** NAC and ellipse of skin also excised

2) Mastectomy with immediate breast reconstruction:

b) **Skin-reducing mastectomy:** NAC excised, Wise pattern incision, majority of skin preserved to accommodate reconstructed breast.
c) **Skin-sparing mastectomy:** NAC excised, entirety of surrounding breast skin preserved for immediate reconstruction.

d) **Nipple-preserving mastectomy:** skin and NAC preserved but underlying breast tissue excised.

Sentinel lymph node biopsy

Figure 4. *Sentinel lymph node biopsy*
See colour centrefold for this image.

A staging procedure often carried out in conjunction with a WLE or mastectomy. A radiolabelled substance such as technetium 99 is injected into the tumour site. A patent blue dye is also then injected on table, before prepping the patient.

'Hot' and blue lymph nodes are theoretically representative of the lymph node in which cancer cells may be taken up if they are to metastasise via lymphatics.

Some centres use intra-operative 'OSNA' analysis to assess for cancer cells within the sentinel lymph node(s). Positive sentinel lymph nodes

Axillary lymph node clearance

Figure 5. *Axillary lymph node biopsy*
See colour centrefold for this image.

Level 1 and 2 lymph nodes are cleared. If clinically involved level 3 nodes are evident, a level 3 clearance can be performed.

The key anatomical landmarks to consider in this procedure include:

- The axillary vein
- Thoracodorsal pedicle
- Long thoracic nerve
- Pectoralis minor (in determining level of clearance)

Therapeutic mammoplasty

An oncoplastic procedure, excising the tumour with a margin of tissue around it, and mobilisation of the remaining breast tissue in order to preserve the breast. This enables breast-conserving excision without leaving significant breast contour deformities.

Figure 6. *Therapeutic mammoplasty*
See colour centrefold for this image.

Breast reduction (symmetrising)

A similar fundamental principle, with most commonly a Wise pattern incision.

Figure 7. *Breast reduction (symmetrising)*
See colour centrefold for this image.

Mastopexy (symmetrising)

Figure 8. *Mastopexy (symmetrising)*
See colour centrefold for this image.

Implant based reconstruction +/- acellular dermal matrix (ADM)

An acellular dermal matric/dermal sling allows additional inferior coverage of an implant during an implant-based reconstruction. This means that if the wound breaks down, the risk of the underlying implant being exposed is reduced.

Figure 9. *Implant based reconstruction +/- acellular dermal matrix*
See colour centrefold for this image.

Section 6: Autologous Breast Reconstruction

Latissimus dorsi

Figure 10. *Latissimus dorsi*
See colour centrefold for this image.

Deep inferior epigastric artery

The deep inferior epigastric artery perforator (DIEP) flap is one of the most important – if not the gold standard of – autologous breast reconstructions.

The breast is reconstructed using a skin paddle and subcutaneous fat from the patient's own abdomen. The flap is based on perforator vessels from the underlying rectus abdominus muscles (i.e. DIEP artery and veins). Post-operatively, the patient will have breast and abdominal wounds.

Figure 11. *Deep inferior epigastric artery reconstruction*
See colour centrefold for this image.

Section 7: How to manage a free flap

As an SHO covering oncoplastic breast patients, you may have to review a free flap, 2-3 times/shift. This is because if a small clot occludes one of the anastomosed vessels, the flap could quickly die. This is a time critical event; the faster the problem is recognised, the higher the chance it can be successfully salvaged in theatre. The risk of such an event is highest in the first hours post-operatively, and depreciates with time after the operation. This is reflected in the frequency of free flap observations.

1) When was the operation done? (This determines the risk of anastomotic problems.)
2) ABCDE assessment, incorporating an assessment of:
    a. Fluid balance
    b. Temperature
3) The flap – is it:
    a. Healthy: Soft, warm, capillary refill time (CRT) 2-3 seconds, good doppler of vessels
    b. Arterial problem: cold, pale, delayed capillary refill, no doppler of arterial phase
    c. Venous problem: congested, swollen, brisk capillary refill
    d. Demarcation: sometimes there is not a problem with the viability of the whole flap (i.e. the vessel anastomosis is patent), but the distal tip appears necrotic.
4) Is there any evidence of a collection? (Breast axilla or abdomen)
5) Drain output. There are usually 2 breast drains and 2 abdominal drains. Drains can be removed as per operation note instructions (e.g. remove when <30mL/24 hours – please be aware drain output temporarily increases once patient starts mobilising so it is best to ask a Senior when they are happy for the drains to be removed).
6) Blood tests:
    a. What is the post-operative Hb? If <8, this may jeopardise flap viability

b. U&Es: copious intraoperative fluids can derange urea and electrolytes.

Key points:

- Importance of a good handover: if you are helping in theatre, ensure your night colleague knows to review the patient. Ideally go with them to show them the flap.
- Importance of seeking Senior support: if you are not experienced at examining free flaps, examine with your SpR. They will want to know if there are any concerns.
- Regular examination: day 0/1 post-op, the flap should be examined at the beginning, middle and end of each shift.

In your plan:

- Document the frequency of flap observations required. This is usually specified in the operation notes (e.g. every 30 minutes for first 12 hours, hourly for the next 6 hours, then 2 hourly for 12 hours, then down to every 4 hours).
- Document need for strict fluid balance
- Prescribe IVI, titrating to BP, HR and UO, particularly if patient is not yet drinking well
- Does the patient need post-op bloods?
- The need for Bairhugger/patient warming device
- VTE – flowtrons, TEDS and timing of LMWH
- If there are concerns, timely escalation to Senior colleague.

CHAPTER 2

EAR, NOSE AND THROAT SURGERY

JESSICA LUNN & RAJ LAKHANI

Abstract

Section 1 – The ENT bag
Section 2 – Useful Examination Techniques
Nasendoscopy
Microscopy
Rennie and Weber Tests
Anterior rhinoscopy
Section 3 – The SOS/EMERGENCY Clinic
Facial nerve palsy
Sudden onset sensorineural hearing loss
Otitis externa
Aural Foreign bodies
Section 4 – The On-call SHO
Ear:
Otitis media and mastoiditis, infection of the pinna, ear trauma including traumatic tympanic membrane perforation, pinna haematoma and pinna lacerations
Nose:
Epistaxis, septal haematomas and abscesses, nasal foreign body, acute rhinosinusitis, periorbital cellulitis
Throat/Neck:
Sore throat, tonsillitis, peritonsillar abscess, parapharyngeal/retropharyngeal abscess, supraglottitis, oropharyngeal malignancy, foreign body, neck lumps, oesophageal food bolus
Section 5 – ENT Emergencies
Stridor
Post-tonsillectomy bleed
Tracheostomies/laryngectomies
Post-thyroidectomy haemorrhage

Abstract

ENT SHO on-call shifts can be initially challenging as they require experience with examination and practical techniques not taught in medical school. This chapter covers how to equip yourself for an ENT shift and details some of the examination skills that are required.

Common emergencies and pathology encountered by an ENT SHO in the emergency clinic and whilst on-call are covered as well as guidance on key features to illicit in history taking, appropriate management and escalation, together with step by step instructions for practical skills.

Section 1: The ENT Bag

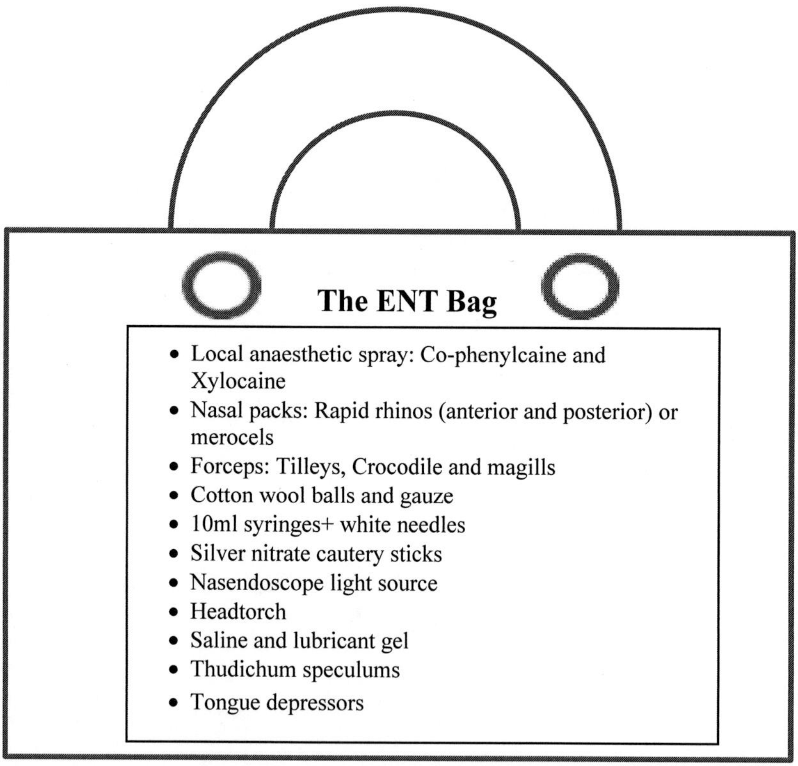

Figure 1. *The ENT bag*

The ENT on-call job is very practical and starting the shift with the necessary equipment packed in one place will make it much easier.

Section 2: Useful examination techniques

Flexible nasendoscopy

Flexible nasendoscopy is used to examine the nasal passages, post nasal space, oropharynx and larynx. Once confident with the technique and after adequate exposure to normal anatomy, it becomes an invaluable tool for the on-call ENT SHO. Figure 2 describes a step by step approach to performing flexible nasendoscopy (Tysome, Kanegaonkar 2012, 33-34). You should initially be supervised until competent.

Flexible nasendoscopy

1. Sign out a scope as per local protocol
2. Explain the procedure to the patient
3. Spray the nose with co-phenylcaine. Warn the patient of the bad taste and not to eat or drink for an hour after use.
4. Clean the end of the scope with an alcohol wipe and ensure it is well focused
5. Apply lubricant gel to the distal part of the scope avoiding the tip
6. Hold the end of the scope with the thumb and index finger, with the middle finger on the patients nose and the eye piece in the other hand
7. Ask the patient to continue breathing
8. Insert the scope into a nostril running it along the floor of the nose (or in between the inferior and middle turbinates)
9. Examine the postnasal space and eustachian tube orifices
10. Ask the patient to breathe in via the nose and angle the scope inferiorly using the control switch
11. Advance the scope into the oropharynx and then larynx
12. Examine the tongue base and vallecula (ask patient to stick out tongue), epiglottis, piriform fossae (ask patient to blow out cheeks), post cricoid regio and supraglottic region
13. Assess the appearance and movement of the vocal cords (ask patient to say 'eeeee')
14. Gently withdraw the scope and explain your findings

Figure 2. *Flexible Nasendoscopy*

Microscopy

Examination of the ear, in addition to otoscopy (not covered in this chapter), using a microscope is often required in clinic or whilst on-call, particularly for performing procedures such as micro-suction or removal of foreign bodies.

Set up the microscope before bringing the patient into the room:

- Adjust the inter-pupillary distance to allow binocular vision
- Adjust the magnification
- Set the refractive power to zero.

Explain the procedure to the patient and ask them to lie supine with their head to one side. Adjust the height of the bed or your chair so that the microscope is level with the patient's ear, then adjust the viewing distance (working distance) to focus the microscope and insert an aural speculum. Use the largest speculum that the ear will admit. Use your middle finger to gently pull the ear posteriorly whilst the speculum is stabilised with the thumb and index finger. Your other hand is free to use suction or instruments under direct vision.

When performing micro-suction use the aural suction tube and suction the wax or debris. Avoid touching the skin of the ear canal to prevent discomfort and trauma. The fine tip suction may be required if the ear canal is very narrow or inflamed. Always warn the patients about the loud noise suction makes to prevent sudden movement and the possibility of dizziness and coughing.

Rinne and Weber test

A simple test to assess hearing, in particular to distinguish between conductive and sensorineural hearing loss. Results should be confirmed with an audiogram.

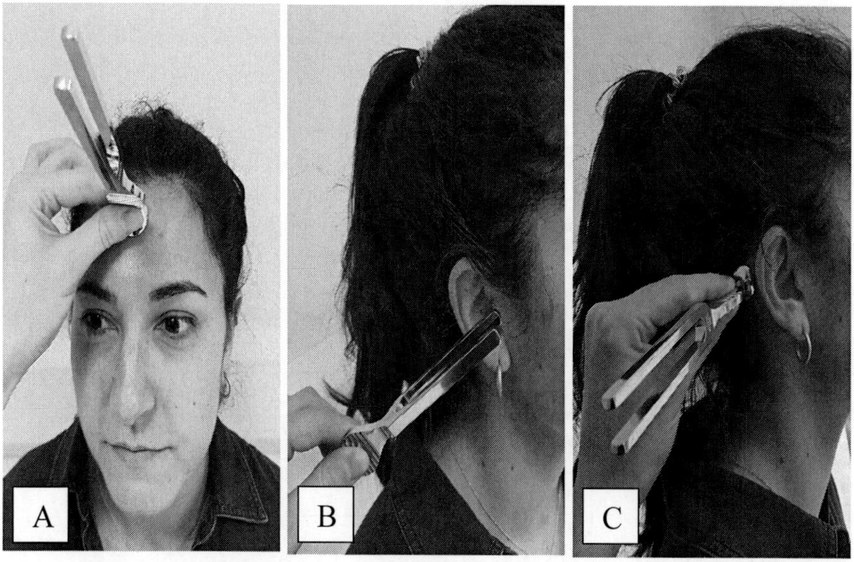

Figure 3. *A) Weber test; B & C) Rinne Tests*

Weber:

- This tests lateralisation of sound via bone conduction.
- Strike a 512Hz tuning fork on your elbow or knee and then place it in the centre of the patient's forehead for up to 4 seconds holding onto the stem (British Society of Audiology 2016).
- Ask whether it is heard louder in the middle or in the left or right ear.
- Patients with normal hearing in both ears will hear it in the middle/centrally.
- If Weber's lateralised to one side, it is helpful to perform Rinne's on this ear first.

Rinne:

- This tests whether air conduction or bone conduction is louder in each ear.
- Place the tines of a resonating 512Hz tuning fork in front of the ear approximately 2.5cm from the external auditory meatus for two seconds. Hold the fork so that the tines are parallel to the ear canal.

Then turn the tuning fork around and firmly press the footplate onto the mastoid for a further two seconds without interrupting the vibrations.

- Ask the patient afterwards whether the sound was louder in front of or behind the ear.
- A positive Rinne's (air conduction louder than bone conduction) is documented when the sound is heard louder in front of the ear.

For interpretation of the tests see Table 1.

	Rinne		
Weber	**Right**	**Left**	**Result**
Central	Positive	Positive	Normal hearing
Lateralises to left	Positive	Positive	Right sensorineural hearing loss
Lateralises to right	Positive	Positive	Left sensorineural hearing loss
Lateralises to left	Positive	Negative	Left conductive hearing loss
Lateralises to right	Negative	Positive	Right conductive hearing loss
Lateralises to left	Negative	Positive	False negative Rinne - severe sensorineural hearing loss right
Lateralises to right	Positive	Negative	False negative Rinne - severe sensorineural hearing loss left

Table 1. *Interpretation of Rinne and Weber tests*

Anterior rhinoscopy

In order to view the anterior nasal cavity, hold a thudichum speculum in your non-dominant hand and a torch in the other hand (if instrumentation is required wear a head torch). Point your index finger towards yourself and hang the metal loop of the speculum over this finger with its prongs facing away. Use your thumb to support the thudichum speculum and place your middle finger and ring finger either side of the speculum (Figure 4a). Gently insert the speculum into each nostril using your middle and ring fingers to open and close it (Figure 4b).

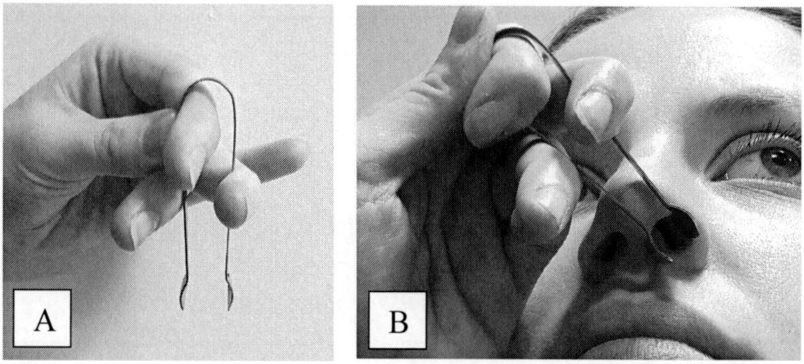

Figure 4. *Anterior rhinoscopy: A) Holding nasal thudichums; B) Anterior rhinoscopy*

Section 3: The SOS/EMERGENCY clinic

Common pathologies seen in ENT Emergency clinic:

- Facial nerve palsy
- Sudden onset sensorineural hearing loss
- Otitis externa
- Ear foreign body
- Nasal Trauma

Facial nerve palsy

Patients will be referred to the emergency clinic by A&E and GPs with a diagnosis of Bell's palsy. Bell's palsy is a diagnosis of exclusion referring to an idiopathic facial nerve palsy in patients whose history and examination are otherwise normal (BMJ Best Practice 2017). During the consultation you will need to take a thorough history and examine the entire course of the facial nerve looking for pathology which may have caused the facial weakness.

Differential Diagnoses of facial nerve palsy

- Upper motor neurone lesions including stroke
- Malignant otitis externa
- Ramsey hunt Syndrome
- Otitis media with facial canal dehiscence or mastoiditis
- Parotid Malignancy
- Traumatic facial nerve palsy (temporal bone fractures)

Figure 5. *Differential diagnosis of facial nerve palsy*

History:

Table 2 highlights the key features to elicit to aid diagnosing idiopathic facial nerve palsy. Patients may also report dysgeusia, xerostomia, eye dryness or hyperlacrimation (De Seta et al. 2014).

	Idiopathic facial nerve palsy	**Think of other pathology**
Onset	Sudden (evolving over up to 72 hours)	Gradually worsening
Course	Gradual improvement over time	Progressive/intermittent /no change
Preceding events	Nil/Viral infection	Trauma/surgery/ear infection
Pain	May have post auricular pain	Otalgia
Hyperacusis	Can be present	Can be present
Ear discharge	Nil	Present
Lumps in parotid/neck	Nil	Present
Systemic features	Nil	Pyrexia/weight loss/fatigue

Table 2. *Idiopathic facial nerve palsy versus other pathology*

Examination:

- Test facial nerve function and document the House Brackman Grading score. Confirm it is a lower motor neurone lesion (forehead not spared).
- Examine the other lower cranial nerves.
- Examine the eye more carefully if eye closure is not intact
- Examine the ear for vesicles, evidence of otitis externa or media.
- Examine the parotid gland for discrete lumps and oral cavity
- Consider hearing tests and acoustic reflex testing.

Management:
The treatment for Bell's palsy is high dose steroids (Prednisolone 1mg/kg up to a maximum of 60mg for 7 days). Consider gastric protection with omeprazole and if the patient is diabetic, advice from the diabetes team may need to be sought or increased frequency of blood sugar monitoring.

Eye protection is important in cases of incomplete eye closure. Preservative free eye drops and ointment are prescribed to prevent the cornea drying and subsequent ulceration. Advise the patient to tape their eye shut at night and refer for urgent outpatient ophthalmology review.

Facial physiotherapy and stretching exercises should be considered early.

Patient discussion and reassurance:
Without treatment approximately 70% of patients' facial nerve function will completely recover and this increases to 85% with treatment (Peitersen 1982, 107-111). This can however take several months and this should be explained to patients early on. Worse prognostic factors include co-morbidities such as diabetes and advanced age. Some improvement in the first 2-3 weeks is good prognostic sign.

Escalation:
Any suspicion of facial nerve palsy post trauma should be discussed immediately. Patients with otitis media or malignant otitis externa require admission and the Registrar should be updated. If there is concern about parotid malignancy refer them to a suspected urgent head and neck cancer clinic but discuss with someone in day time hours so that appropriate investigations such as ultrasound guided fine needle aspiration and MRI can be arranged.

Ramsey Hunt syndrome

This is a reactivation of Herpes Zoster virus in the geniculate ganglion of the facial nerve. It is characterised by otalgia, a vesicular rash of the external ear and canal and facial nerve palsy. It may also involve the vestibulocochlear nerve causing sensorineural hearing loss. Vesicles may be seen on the palate and buccal mucosa. The treatment is the same as for Bell's palsy plus a course of oral acyclovir. Admission is only required if there is secondary cellulitis of the external ear.

Sudden onset sensorineural hearing loss (SSNHL)

In practice this term is mainly used to describe an idiopathic sudden onset unilateral sensorineural hearing loss. Current theories for the cause of this include viral inflammation or a vascular insult to the inner ear. Some departments have a specific protocol in place for these patients, so follow this if available. As a general rule treat this as an emergency and when taking referrals, organise for the patient to be seen within 24 hours when audiometry is available but advise upon starting oral steroid treatment by the referring clinician (Figure 6).

SSNHL Top tips

- GP's will often explain results of Rinne and Weber tests over the phone so ensure you have a good understanding of the interpretation of these tests
- SSNHL can have a significant impact on patients' lives- discuss these concerns

Figure 6. *Top tips for SSNHL*

History:
Confirm a history of SSNHL which is usually unilateral and occurs suddenly, or over a few hours. Ask about associated symptoms such as tinnitus, vertigo and pain. Identify any other possible causes of sudden sensorineural hearing loss (Figure 7 - Warner et al 2009, 468).

Acquired Causes of Sensorineural loss

- Iatrogenic – Recent ear surgery
- Trauma – temporal bone fracture
- Infective – such as meningitis
- Loud noise exposure
- Drugs – ototoxic
- Autoimmune – Wegners granulomatosis
- Neoplastic – Acoustic neuroma
- Neurological – cerebrovascular events

Figure 7. *Acquired Causes of sensorineural hearing loss*

Examination:
Perform otoscopy to rule out common causes of conductive hearing loss including wax impaction, otitis media and externa and tympanic membrane perforation. Next, organise an urgent pure tone audiogram and tympanometry or initially perform Rinne and Weber tests if audiogram is unavailable.

Management:
Start high dose steroids (1mg/kg prednisolone, maximum 60mg once daily) for seven days if an audiogram is consistent with new SSNHL or if otoscopy is unremarkable with a convincing history and Rinne and Weber test until an audiogram can be obtained. Follow up is recommended in otology clinic for consideration of intra-tympanic steroids if required and an MRI of the internal acoustic meatus to rule out cerebellopontine pathology such as a vestibular schwannoma. Studies have shown up to 4% of patients presenting with SSNHL have a vestibular schwannoma (Lee, Lee, Hwang 2011, 75-78).

Patient explanation:
In most cases the cause of the hearing loss is not identified. Studies have varying results but approximately 50-60% of patients' hearing will recover (Weinaug 1984, 346-351; Heiden, Porzsolt, Biesinger, Höing 2000, 621-623). Ask patients to seek immediate advice if the other ear becomes affected. Worse prognostic factors include dizziness at presentation, co-morbidities (e.g. diabetes) and advanced age.

Otitis externa

Otitis externa is a common and painful condition where the external ear canal becomes infected and inflamed. Whilst on-call you will receive many referrals from both GPs and A&E about patients with painful discharging ears and muffled hearing.

If referred from a GP and patient is systemically well with no spreading cellulitis they do not need to be seen the same day and can be seen in the emergency clinic, but should be initiated on topical antibiotic drops.

Red flags/Risk factors for malignant otitis externa

- Infection refractory to several weeks of topical treatment
- Elderly diabetic/immunocompromised patients/immunosuppressant drugs
- Pain waking patient at night
- Facial nerve palsy or other cranial nerve involvement
- Granulation tissue/bone exposed on examination of EAC

Figure 8. *Red flags for malignant otitis externa*

History:
Key precipitating factors in the history include foreign bodies in the ear, including use of cotton buds, regular swimming and flaring of skin conditions including eczema and psoriasis.

Elicit red flags to help distinguish between a simple otitis externa versus malignant otitis externa which occurs when the infection has spread from the ear canal leading to osteomyelitis of the skull base (Figure 8)

Examination:
Examine the ear with a microscope or otoscope. The external ear canal will be swollen and inflamed, often containing white/yellow discharge and debris obscuring the tympanic membrane. It is good practice to take a swab which can be used to direct further treatment if required.

Ensure the external ear is also examined to rule out infection spreading to the pinna and examine the cranial nerves in particular the facial nerve as this is most commonly affected in malignant otitis externa.

Otitis Externa – Top tips

- If the canal contains spores/black spots think fungal not bacterial and treat accordingly. These patients will require regular micro-suction and prolonged topical anti-fungal treatment.
- Always check blood sugars in diabetic patients and ensure good control to improve infection recovery
- Encourage patients not to itch their ears with anything particularly not cotton buds and keep their ears dry

Figure 9. *Otitis Externa Top Tips*

Management:
Patients with otitis externa do not usually need to be admitted to hospital **unless there is high suspicion of malignant otitis externa or spreading cellulitis**.

Treat them with topical antibiotics/anti-fungals (Figure 10) for at least one-week, micro-suction of the debris and good analgesia. If the canal is very swollen, a small sponge called a "pope wick" can be inserted into the canal to facilitate the passage of the drops (Figure 10). These patients need to be reviewed again in 48 hours to remove the pope wick.

Oral antibiotics are not indicated in uncomplicated otitis externa unless it is secondary to an otitis media that has perforated through the tympanic membrane, or if there is spreading cellulitis to the pinna (in which case admission may be needed). Be careful using ototoxic drops (gentamicin or neomycin) in patients with perforations or grommets. If they are required, do not use them for more than 1-2 weeks (Phillips 2000, 330-336).

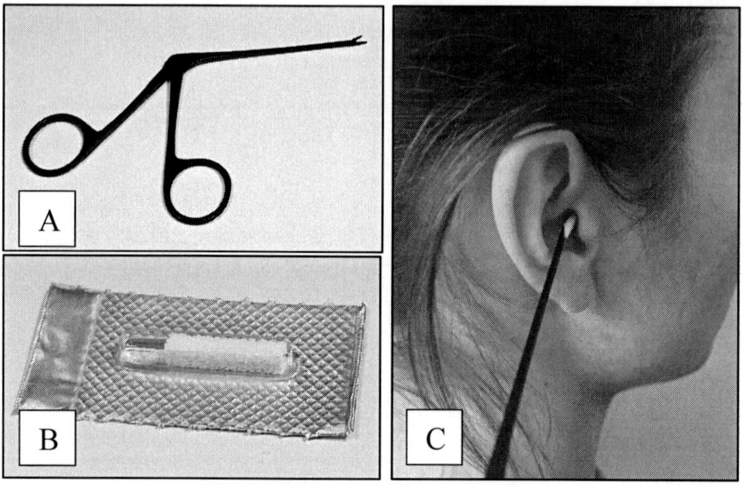

Figure 10. *A) crocodile forceps B) pope wick C) pope wick insertion*

Commonly used topical treatments for otitis externa

- Sofradex drops
- Gentisone HC drops
- Clotrimazole drops
- Ofloxacin drops
- Ciprofloxacin drops

Figure 11. *Topical treatment for otitis externa*

Patients with suspected malignant otitis externa should be admitted and undergo imaging (CT temporal bones or MRI), be started on intravenous and topical antibiotics, as per local policy and have regular micro-suction.

Aural Foreign bodies

Foreign bodies in the ear range from insects and cotton buds in adults to beads and stickers in children. This is not an emergency and the object does not need to be removed that day unless it is an organic foreign body or **a button battery** which are corrosive and can cause necrosis of skin and bone (Premachandra, MrRae 1990, 52-53).

Foreign bodies should be removed under the microscope if available. Useful instruments include micro-suction, wax hooks, Jobson Horne probes and crocodile forceps, depending on the nature of the object. Care must be taken not to cause trauma to the ear canal or tympanic membrane especially in children who may not sit still. If removal is not successful in a child they will require a short general anaesthetic. They can go home and be discussed with a Senior and put on an appropriate list. If there is trauma to an ear canal, often a short course (5 days) of topical antibiotics is prescribed and patients are advised about the symptoms of infection including pain and discharge.

Aural Foreign bodies - Top Tips

- If a child has had multiple attempts to remove a foreign body in the emergency department don't keep trying that day as they will be distressed, bring them back to a clinic another day.
- Ensure the parents agree with attempts at removal without anaesthesia. It is sensible to have a nurse to accompany you.
- Explanation and positioning of the chid is key. It is good practice to ask the parents to hold the child whilst attempting removal.

Figure 12. *Aural Foreign bodies Top Tips*

Nasal trauma

This is commonly seen in the emergency clinic and the SHO on-call also often receives phone calls about fractured nasal bones. These patients do not need to be seen acutely during an on-call unless there is significant epistaxis or a suspected septal haematoma. They should be followed up in 5-7 days post injury to assess the nasal bones once the swelling has reduced.

History:
Key features include the timing and mechanism of the injury. Ask about sense of smell, symptoms of nasal obstruction and rule out CSF rhinorrhoea. Screen for other injuries such as C-spine injuries and enquire about double vision. Ascertain whether the patient feels their nose has changed shape from prior to the injury.

Examination:
Examine the nose from above and behind the patient to look for deviation of the nasal bones and the septum for deviation and septal haematoma. In addition, with high impact injuries assess the periorbital region for ridges, tenderness, loss of infra-orbital sensation and assess eye movements. If you suspect a **septal haematoma** use co-phenylcaine spray to reduce any swelling and palpate the swelling for fluctuance.

Management:
Imaging is not required for nasal injuries unless other facial fractures are suspected. If there is new nasal bone deviation and the patient would like an attempt at manipulation under general or local anaesthesia, list them for this within 2 weeks of the injury before the nasal bones become fixed. A suspected septal haematoma will require prompt formal drainage and therefore will need to be discussed with your Registrar or Consultant.

Patient explanation/Reassurance:
Reassure the patient that nasal fractures do not require any formal treatment and manipulation is to improve the appearance of the nose if indicated and desired. Warn the patient that the nose may not look exactly the same as pre-injury after manipulation. If they have significant septal deviation and this causes symptoms of nasal obstruction in the future they can be referred by their GP in three to four months for consideration of a septoplasty or septorhinoplasty, if required. Manipulation of the nose under anaesthesia is unlikely to improve a blocked nose caused by a new septal deflection.

Section 4: The On-call SHO

Ear

Otitis media

Otitis media is usually managed by general practitioners with antipyretics and oral antibiotics. However, serious complications can occur (Figure 13) and if there is any suspicion of such a complication the patient is referred to ENT.

A common referral to the on-call SHO is to rule out mastoiditis in a child with otitis media. Acute mastoiditis is an inflammatory process involving the mucosa of the mastoid air cells and can rarely lead to sub periosteal abscess formation. Suspect this in an **unwell, pyrexic child with pain over the mastoid area**. The ear may be displaced antero-inferiorly with tender boggy, erythematous post-auricular swelling. Many referrals seen are not mastoiditis and differentials include otitis media with perforation and secondary otitis externa (treat with topical antibiotic drops in addition to oral antibiotics), or post-auricular lymph nodes.

Complications of Otitis Media

Extra-cranial
Intra-temporal
Facial nerve palsy
Mastoiditis/mastoid abscess
Sensorinerual hearing loss
Dizziness
Extra-temporal
Septicaemia
Bezold/Lucs/Citelli abscess

Intra-cranial
Meningitis
Intracranial/epidural/subdural abscesses
Sigmoid/lateral Sinus thrombosis

Figure 13. *Complication of Otitis Media*

However, if mastoiditis is suspected inform seniors and start the child on broad spectrum intravenous antibiotics. They may subsequently require a CT brain and temporal bones and cortical mastoidectomy with grommet insertion depending on clinical progress with antibiotics.

Infection of the pinna

This includes pinna cellulitis, perichondritis (infection of the cartilage) and pinna abscesses. Have a low threshold for admitting patients with an erythematous, hot, tender pinna for intravenous antibiotics as compromise to the cartilage can lead to permanent deformity of ear shape.

History:
Ask about aetiological factors including recent piercings, bites, trauma and otitis externa (pain and discharge). If they have had recurrent episodes or

have a history of rheumatological disease consider relapsing perichondritis as a differential diagnosis.

Examination:
Sparing of the lobule suggests a perichondritis rather than a cellulitis. Palpate for any areas of fluctuance to rule out abscess or haematoma. Examine the external ear canal for signs of otitis externa.

Management:
Treat with intravenous antibiotics as per local microbiology guidelines. If caused by otitis externa, ensure Pseudomonas cover and add in topical antibiotics. All earrings should be removed from the affected ear and any abscesses should be drained promptly. This can often be done under local anaesthetic (Figure 14) for adults; however, children will require a general anaesthetic.

Figure 14. *A) Normal ear anatomy B) Pinna block*
See colour centrefold for this image.

Ear trauma

Referrals can range from advice about temporal bone fractures to straight forward tympanic membrane perforations and pinna lacerations. Patients with temporal bone fractures often have concurrent brain injury and are looked after by trauma or neurosurgical teams. When asked to review these patients it is vital to establish early whether they have any immediate facial nerve palsy at the time of injury as this may require urgent intervention. Delayed presentation of facial nerve palsy is treated with oral high dose steroids as likely due to oedema. Otherwise the care of their brain injury takes precedence and they can be managed in otology outpatients following audiogram. These patients also often have a haemotympanum and lacerations in the external ear canal which may affect their hearing and are usually managed conservatively.

Traumatic tympanic membrane perforation

Direct blows to the pinna may cause sudden pain, hearing loss and bloody discharge. Examination reveals a hole in the tympanic membrane often with bleeding edges. Document the location and whether the perforation is central/marginal and re-assure the patient that most perforations heal over several months with return to normal hearing. Patients can be followed up by their GP and if they have a residual perforation of the tympanic membrane they can be referred back to ENT. Advise all patients to keep their ears dry to prevent recurrent infection.

Pinna haematoma

A haematoma between the cartilage and perichondrium requires prompt drainage to prevent disruption of the blood supply to the cartilage and subsequent necrosis and deformity (Figure 15).

Figure 15. *Incision of pinna haematoma*
See colour centrefold for this image.

Drainage of Pinna Haematoma

1. Perform an ear block
2. Prep the ear with betadine
3. Make an incision under and along the helical rim (for best cosmesis) – Fig. 15.
4. Express the haematoma through the incision
5. Wash out with saline
6. Leave incision open
7. Apply compression with through and through mattress suture through dental rolls/sialastic splints/soaked cotton wool either side of the ear. Cut and shape splints to the area to be compressed

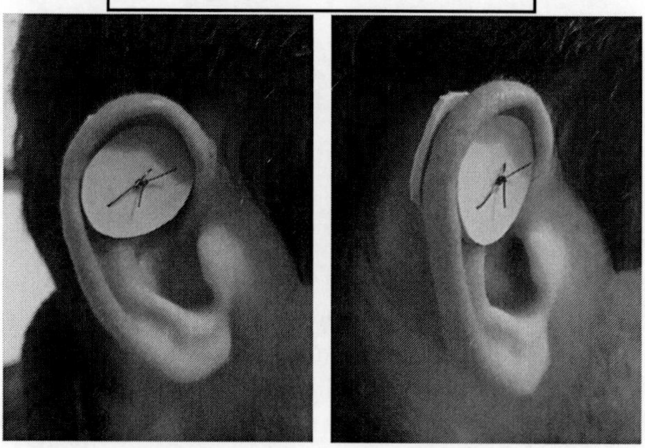

Figure 16. *Drainage of pinna haematoma and compression using sialastic splints following drainage of pinna haematoma*

These usually occur as a result of blunt trauma often related to sports such as boxing or rugby and present as a painful swelling of the pinna. Following aspiration or drainage give the patient 7 days of oral antibiotics (co-amoxiclav) and arrange for them to return for review in 48 hours. Advise patients not to take part in contact sports for 4-6 weeks to prevent re-accumulation of the haematoma.

Pinna lacerations

These can be cleaned and repaired in adults under local anaesthetic. Use non-absorbable interrupted sutures (such as a 5.0/6.0 prolene/nylon) to oppose skin edges and ensure underlying cartilage is covered. Cartilage may also need to be repaired first with interrupted absorbable sutures (such as 5.0 vicryl) or trimmed in cases of skin loss where the skin does not approximate. It is advisable to cover patients with broad spectrum antibiotics such as co-amoxiclav for one week.

Nose

Epistaxis

Epistaxis is one of the most commonly encountered pathologies as an SHO on-call. Most cases of epistaxis can be managed conservatively in the emergency department and discharged. However, some will require packing and admitting under ENT.

History:

Key points to elicit in the history include:

- Time of onset
- Duration
- Precipitating factors
- Side of the nose of onset
- Anterior vs posterior (initially coming from the front of the nose or running down the back of the throat)
- Risk or aetiologic factors (Figure 17)
- Red flags for sinonasal malignancy

Often patients with profuse epistaxis are elderly and taking anticoagulants so information about why they are on these drugs, recent INRs, other past medical history and who they live with at home, are all vital parts of the history. It is also important is to elicit any objections to receiving blood products if required (e.g. Jehovah Witness community) and if there are objections, then discussion with haematologists and relevant representatives may be required.

Risk Factors/Underlying Aetiology of Epistaxis

- Uncontrolled hypertension
- Anticoagulants
- Recent trauma (including nose picking or foreign body)
- Prolonged use of oxygen via nasal cannulae/nasal CPAP
- Known haematological disorders – thrombocytopenia/HHT/haemophilia
- Nasopharyngeal/sinonasal tumours
- Recent nasal/sinus surgery

Figure 17. *Risk Factors/ Underlying Aetiology of Epistaxis*

Examination:
On arrival in the emergency department often the bleeding has already been controlled by the staff there and the patient has nasal packing in situ. In this scenario, examination should include visualisation of the other side of the nose and the oropharynx to ensure bleeding is not ongoing.

If the patient has not already been managed as above, perform an ABCDE assessment, apply compression to the front of the nose and ice packs to the neck/forehead. Use a thudichums speculum and headlight to examine the anterior septum looking for bleeding points. Using small cotton wool balls soaked in co-phenylcaine (otherwise known as blue spray), placed on the septum using crocodile forceps may help to clean the septum, anaesthetise and allow bleeding points to be visualised.

Management:

- Cautery – Patients who have bleeding from the anterior septum (Little's area) can be cauterised with silver nitrate sticks. This should be attempted before packing to avoid unnecessary packing and admission. As above, use thudichums, a head torch and co-phenylcaine (which acts as a topical anaesthetic) and then under direct vision, apply silver nitrate around and over the vessel, covering as small an area as possible to stop the bleeding.

If the bleeding is controlled, keep the patient in the emergency department for a period of observation and then discharge them. Avoid cauterisation on both sides of the septum due to the risk of necrosis and perforation. Advise patients to avoid strenuous activity/lifting, nose picking/blowing and steaming hot food and drinks.

Epistaxis Top Tips

- Always wear personal protective gear – gloves/gown/mask with visor and have suction available
- Avoid packing in patients with hereditary haemorrhagic telengectasia /thrombocytopaenia (causes more trauma and further bleeding) and gain senior and haematology advice. If packing must be used, use a soft dissolvable pack such as nasopore.
- If bleeding continues despite packing with rapid rhino check sufficient air inflation of balloon (see guidance on pack)
- Don't underestimate uncontrolled hypertension, treat early and ask for medical help if needed.
- Look out for repeated swallowing in children/patients who are unable to communicate – red flag for posterior bleeding
- Be –aware of patients with COPD who may de-saturate with nasal packs in situ
- Always ask about peanut allergies before using naseptin cream (contains peanut oil)

Figure 18. *Epistaxis management top tips*

- Packing – If compression and cauterisation fail, a nasal pack will be required. Commonly used packs include merocels (expand by soaking with sterile water once in situ) and rapid rhinos (inflated using air balloons – Figure 19). Rapid rhinos come in different sizes for anterior and posterior packing. Start by using an anterior pack on the side where the bleeding originated. If this fails to control the bleeding insert a pack on the other side. If the bleeding does not settle and the balloons are adequately inflated, remove these packs and use posterior packs (either a posterior double balloon rapid rhino or a Foley catheter, depending on availability and the unit you are working in).

Once inserted, nasal packs are usually kept in for at least 24 hours before removal, if bleeding is controlled. The patient is usually admitted to hospital for this period. If they are kept in for more than 24-48 hours the patient should be covered with oral antibiotics to prevent infection.

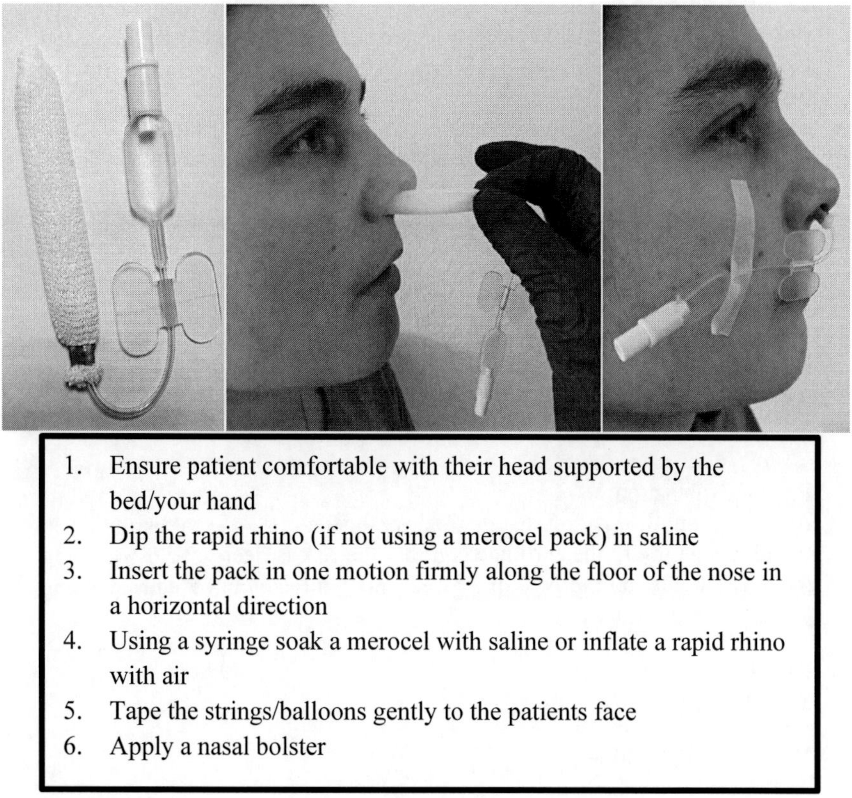

1. Ensure patient comfortable with their head supported by the bed/your hand
2. Dip the rapid rhino (if not using a merocel pack) in saline
3. Insert the pack in one motion firmly along the floor of the nose in a horizontal direction
4. Using a syringe soak a merocel with saline or inflate a rapid rhino with air
5. Tape the strings/balloons gently to the patients face
6. Apply a nasal bolster

Figure 19. *Anterior Nasal Packing. Illustration and step wise approach*

- Surgery – If packing fails, vessel ligation may be required, most commonly sphenopalatine artery ligation. Contact Seniors early and prepare the patient for theatre.

Septal haematomas and abscesses

History:
Suspect a septal haematoma or abscess in a patient presenting with nasal pain, symptoms of obstruction or fever post nasal trauma, or nasal surgery such as septoplasty.

Examination:
Examine the septum looking for a tender, compressible/fluctuant/boggy septal swelling. Septal haematomas are often described as bilateral cherry red swellings. Blood or pus has collected between the septal cartilage and the mucoperichondrium (within which the blood supply runs) (Ambrus et al. 1981, 575-582). If not promptly drained ischaemia of the cartilage may occur leading to deformity of the nose (Canty, Berkowitz 1996, 1373-1376; Ketcham, Han 2010, 897-904). In addition, it is important to be aware of the possibility of intracranial complications of abscesses, such as cavernous sinus thrombosis.

Management:
All patients suspected to have a septal haematoma or abscess should be discussed with Seniors, admitted, started on IV antibiotics, made NBM and taken to theatre for incision and drainage under general anaesthetic. If a septal abscess is suspected and the patient is having fevers, then a contrast enhanced CT scan should be ordered to assess their cavernous sinus.

Patient explanation:
Explain about the risk of change in shape of the nose due to disruption in the blood supply to the cartilage and that the risk is decreased by draining the haematoma promptly. An abscess may already have caused some cartilage destruction.

Figure 20. *Septal haematoma*
See colour centrefold for this image.

Nasal Foreign bodies

Nasal foreign bodies most commonly occur in children and need to be removed that day, or the subsequent day in theatre, as they pose a potential risk to the airway (Figure 21). Examine the nose using thudichums, or an otoscope to confirm foreign body. The first thing to try is the 'mother's kiss' (Purohit, Ray, Wilson, Chawla 2008, 420-422) which involves the parent blowing into the child's mouth whilst the nostril without the foreign body is occluded. If this is not successful, attempt removal of the foreign body with a Jobson Horne probe, hook or crocodile forceps depending what it is.

If this is not successful book the child for removal under general anaesthetic. If this cannot be done the same day seek advice from Seniors to decide whether the child should be admitted or could go home and return the following morning.

Nasal Foreign Bodies - Top tips

- Jobson Horne probes work very well for beads in the nose
- Always consider foreign body in a child presenting with unilateral smelly nasal discharge
- You often only have one chance so ensure you have the appropriate help and equipment
- Always warn parents there may be some mild bleeding
- Help and positioning of the child is imperative for successful removal. Enlist the help of a nurse and ensure the parents are happy to hold the child firmly to help removal.

Figure 21. *Nasal Foreign Bodies*

Figure 22. *Jobson Horne Probe*
See colour centrefold for this image.

Acute Rhinosinusitis

Sinusitis is not usually seen whilst on-call as is managed in the community, however it is important to be familiar with the acute complications including peri-orbital cellulitis and intracranial spread of infection causing meningitis, abscesses and sinus thrombosis. Have a high suspicion for acute fulminant fungal sinusitis in an un-well immunocompromised patient with sinusitis and neurological signs.

Periorbital cellulitis

This should be managed jointly by paediatrics, ENT and ophthalmology and is considered an ENT emergency as optic nerve compression may lead to irreversible blindness. Infection spreads from the ethmoid sinuses, through lamina papyracea and into the orbit. This can lead to sub periosteal and orbital abscesses which require urgent drainage. Discuss all these patients with a Senior.

History:
Elicit a history of upper respiratory tract infection versus insect bites/cuts.

Examination:
The periorbital region will be erythematous, swollen and tender. Examine the nose for evidence of inflamed mucosa and mucopus. Examine the eye for proptosis, chemosis, pain/double vision on eye movement, abnormal visual acuity, and colour vision. Drowsiness and vomiting should raise suspicion of intracranial involvement.

Management:
Admit all patients for intravenous antibiotics, topical nasal treatment (nasal steroids, saline nasal douches and xylometazoline drops) and daily ophthalmology review.

If any eye signs are elicited, there is suspicion of sub periosteal abscess, or there is no clinical improvement with antibiotics, an urgent CT sinuses and orbit should be arranged with subsequent urgent drainage of any abscess in theatre (open or endoscopic).

Throat/Neck

Sore throat

This is a very common presentation seen on an ENT on-call and most often involves management of tonsillitis, glandular fever or peritonsillar abscesses, however, it is important to be able to spot other possible diagnoses (Figure 23). **Top Tip**: If ever in doubt about the pathology – the patient requires flexible nasendoscopy

Sore Throat - Other Diagnoses to Consider

- Supraglottitis/epiglottitis
- Parapharyngeal abscess
- Retropharyngeal abscess
- Aerodigestive tract foreign body
- Oropharyngeal/laryngeal malignancy

Figure 23. *Sore Throat differential diagnosis*

Tonsillitis

History:
Young patients with sore throat, odynophagia and fever with bilateral or unilateral enlarged erythematous/exudative tonsils. Establish whether they can eat and drink and whether they have already tried oral antibiotics. Patients with glandular fever have similar symptoms with fatigue and muscle aches and large bilateral cervical lymphadenopathy.

Management:

- Ensure bloods (FBC, CRP U&E, LFTS and monospot) have been taken.
- Can be managed as an outpatient unless unable to tolerate fluids or oral antibiotics.
- Treat with IV benzypenicillin 1.2g 4 hourly (clarithroymin in penicillin allergy) if IV antibiotics required
- ± IV fluids and analgesia (including difflam mouthwash/spray)
- Some may benefit from a dose of IV dexamethasone 8mg.
- These patients usually require only 24 hours treatment and are discharged once able to eat and drink. If they have recurrent tonsillitis, recommend they be referred by their GP to ENT clinic for consideration of tonsillectomy (see Figure 24 – NHS Quality improvement Scotland 2010).

SIGN Criteria for Tonsillectomy

- 7+ well documented, clinically significant, adequately treated sore throats in the preceding year

OR

- 5+ episodes in each of the preceding two years

OR

- 3+ episodes in each of the preceding three years.

Figure 24. *Criteria for Tonsillectomy* (The Scottish Intercollegiate Guidelines Network)

Glandular fever is treated the same as tonsillitis but advise patients not to take part in contact sports for 8 weeks due to the risk of splenic rupture (Bartlett, Williams, Hilton 2016, 531-538).

Peritonsillar abscess

History:
The sore throat is worse on one side, they often cannot swallow even saliva and have an altered voice (hot potato voice). Examination is difficult due to trismus and they may have stertor. On one side the anterior arch will be erythematous and pushed medially with deviation of the uvula to the opposite side and a bulging palate.

Figure 25. *A) Normal Oropharynx B) Tonsillitis C) Peritonsillar abscess*
See colour centrefold for this image.

Management:

Be aware that these patients can have airway compromise. If the airway is safe, treat as per tonsillitis with the addition of IV metronidazole, IV dexamethasone 8mg and needle aspiration or incision and drainage (Figure 26). If they have trismus it can be very helpful for visualisation to give good analgesia and dexamethasone before attempting drainage. Peritonsillar erythema and oedema with no pus is diagnosed as peritonsillar cellulitis.

Figure 26. *Peritonsillar abscess drainage*
See colour centrefold for this image.

Parapharyngeal/retropharyngeal abscess

The clinical features of parapharyngeal abscess can include:

- Sore throat
- Dysphagia
- Pyrexia
- Unilateral neck swelling
- Trismus
- Limited neck movements.

Examination of the oropharynx may also show medialisation of the tonsil. In suspected abscesses flexible nasendoscopy should be performed and can show bulging (medial displacement) of the lateral pharyngeal wall.

Retropharyngeal abscesses are more common in children. Suspect an abscess in an unwell child with a recent URTI who is refusing to eat or drink and is holding their head to one side, or has neck stiffness. They can also present with airway compromise. Flexible nasendoscopy may show bulging of the posterior pharyngeal wall.

Management:

- Ensure the airway is safe.
- In severe cases tracheostomy may be required.
- Lateral soft tissue neck X-ray can help diagnose retropharyngeal abscesses, but CT neck is required to confirm a collection and plan for any surgical drainage. Discuss any children with a Senior before ordering this.
- Resuscitate all septic patients including starting IV antibiotics.
- Keep them nil by mouth until Senior review.
- If drainage is required this can be done orally or via the neck depending on the abscess.

Supraglottitis

A patient with a severe sore throat and a normal oropharynx should have an urgent flexible nasendoscopy and be discussed with a Senior. Other features include a hoarse voice, fever, drooling and stridor.

Management:

- Contact Seniors immediately and depending on severity they may need urgent anaesthetic review and securing of airway with intubation or tracheostomy.
- They require care in ITU, HDU or a specific airway bed on an ENT ward and **should be moved to resus** if still in the A&E department.
- Treat with high flow oxygen or heliox if available
- Regular IV dexamethasone 8mg (three times daily), adrenaline nebulisers (1ml of 1 in 1000 diluted in saline) and IV antibiotics (e.g. ceftriaxone – refer to local guidelines).

Oropharyngeal malignancy

Suspect this in an older patient presenting with unilateral sore throat with a longer history and significant risk factors (such as smoking and alcohol (squamous cell carcinoma) or a patient with unilateral large tonsil with night sweats and weight loss (lymphoma).

Treat for infection as appropriate including ensuring the airway is safe. Discuss with Seniors to arrange urgent head and neck follow up as an outpatient if they can tolerate food and drink orally.

Foreign body

Fish bones and other foreign bodies often become stuck in a tonsil or the tongue base. Using a headlight, tongue depressor look very carefully as they can be well hidden and can look like saliva. Also palpate the tongue base and tonsils gently with a gloved finger after application of local anaesthesic spray. A bone is occasionally palpable if not visible.

Using co-phenylcaine spray can help and use forceps such as Tilley's to remove the foreign body. If visible further down (such as the tongue base) on flexible nasendoscopy it may still be possible to remove them orally using Magills forceps under scope guidance with assistance from another person. However, they may require removal under general anaesthetic.

If there is a strong history of foreign body including odynophagia and dysphagia and the patient is able to point to specific location in the neck, but it isn't visible, further investigation should include a lateral soft tissue

X-ray and then a CT neck (deemed more useful than x-ray with fish bones (Lue, Fang, Manolidis 2000, 435-438), or examination under anaesthetic.

Admit these patients, discuss with a Senior, start IV fluids and keep them nil by mouth.

Neck Lumps

Acute neck lumps seen whilst on-call are often infective in nature. In adults the differential diagnoses include:

- Deep neck space abscesses (see sore throat section)
- Infected sebaceous cysts
- Reactive lymphadenopathy
- Submandibular or parotid swellings (see sialadenitis section).
- Consider haematomas in post-surgical or traumatic cases.

Infected subcutaneous cysts require incision and drainage usually under local anaesthetic with wick insertion and oral antibiotics. If the swelling appears cystic but deeper, organise an USS scan (+/- aspiration) as occasionally adults can present with infected branchial or thyroglossal cysts. This is much more common in children and they often require admission for IV antibiotics.

Lymphadenitis is a common cause of a large tender neck swelling in children. The overlying skin may be erythematous. If well, they may be treated with oral antibiotics. However, if not improving on oral antibiotics or are unwell, they require admission for IV antibiotics. Occasionally this may progress to abscess formation and if suspected perform a neck ultrasound.

Oesophageal Food Bolus

With all ingested foreign bodies, it is vital to elicit whether they are sharp or not, including if food eaten could have contained any bones.

Soft

In some units lower oesophageal food boluses (below the suprasternal notch) are managed by gastroenterology and high boluses by ENT, however there is an increasing trend towards all soft boluses being managed by gastroenterology with flexible endoscopy.

Check the local policy before accepting patients and ascertain in the history if the patient has had repeated episodes as this may indicate a stricture or malignancy that requires gastroenterology follow up.

History/Examination:
Soft food boluses present as sudden onset discomfort and aphagia/dysphagia following a meal. They are often spitting out their own saliva or retching. With high obstruction (commonly at the level of cricopharyngeus) the patient points to discomfort in the neck and has immediate regurgitation with a trial sip of water. Flexible nasendoscopy will show pooling of the saliva in the hypopharynx.

Management:

- These patients should be admitted for observation, optimal analgesia and IV fluids.
- Various medical treatments to help relieve the obstruction have been suggested with limited evidence, including a dose of diazepam and serial doses of 20mg IV buscopan.
- If there is no resolution of symptoms later that day, or the following morning, a flexible endoscopy by gastroenterology, or rigid oesophagoscopy by ENT is indicated.
- If there is any concern of airway compromise suggested by stridor, shortness of breath or voice change, inform a Senior immediately and obtain an anaesthetic review.

Sharp

Sharp oesophageal foreign bodies should be treated as an emergency due to the risk of oesophageal perforation. Features in the history and examination suggestive of this include severe chest and back pain, presence of surgical emphysema, tachypnoea and tachycardia. If the patient does not have signs of perforation following examination, perform a lateral soft tissue neck X-ray and chest X-ray, make them NBM and contact Seniors. Corrosive foreign bodies should be treated in a similar fashion and removed urgently e.g. button batteries.

Sialadenitis

Patients may present to ENT with painful, swollen salivary glands. Acutely this is usually related to inflammation/infection with or without obstruction and more commonly affects the parotid gland.

Parotitis

Elderly, dehydrated patients with co-morbidities or poor oral hygiene are particularly susceptible to parotitis. They usually present with tender swelling over the parotid region and difficulty eating and drinking. Examine the pre-auricular area, the neck and the oral cavity including an attempt to express pus from the parotid duct. Most patients can be managed with conservative treatment including hydration, analgesia, sialogogues (such as lemon sweets), warm compresses and oral antibiotics if required.

If they are systemically unwell, there is fluctuant swelling suggestive of an abscess, spreading cellulitis of the overlying skin or they are unable to drink anything, admission is required for IV antibiotics and fluids. Arrange an ultrasound and drainage as appropriate for suspected abscesses. As elderly patients with an acute parotitis often have an underlying medical cause, care under the medical team may be appropriate.

Submandibular sialadenitis

Patients present with pain and swelling to one of the submandibular glands which is worse when eating and drinking.

The general treatment and admission criteria are the same as for parotitis above. Of note, swelling in the submandibular region may be related to dental infection or abscess and therefore as well as bimanual palpation of the floor of the mouth for salivary stones, palpation of the teeth should be included in the examination. If dental pathology is suspected, an orthopantomogram (OPG) should be performed and a dental opinion obtained.

Outpatient follow up of suspected stones or strictures should be arranged for when acute infections have settled.

Section 5: ENT Emergencies

Stridor

Attend to patients with reported stridor immediately. There are many different causes of stridor in the acute setting (Figure 27).

Differential Diagnoses of Acute Stridor

Adult
Infective: Supraglottitis, deep space neck abscess
Traumatic: Laryngeal trauma
Malignant: Laryngeal tumour with critical obstruction
Iatrogenic: Post-operative neck haematoma, bilateral vocal cord palsy
Psychogenic: Paradoxical cord movement,
Other: Foreign body, anaphylaxis

Paediatric
Infective: Viral croup, epiglottis, retropharyngeal/parapharyngeal abscess, tracheitis
Other: foreign body inhalation

Figure 27. *Differential Diagnosis of Acute Stridor*

Definitive management depends on the cause. However, the following initial management strategies are important to put in place before Senior help arrives (Figure 28).

Initial Management of An Acutely Stridulous Patient

- Ensure the patient is in a suitable environment, such as resus
- Perform an initial bed side assessment of the airway and try to keep the patient as calm as possible.
  Questions
  - Is it true stridor or stertor (low pitched snoring)/wheeze (polyphonic expiratory sounds)?
  - Is the stridor inspiratory (supraglottic), expiratory (tracheobronchial) or biphasic?
  - Is the patient compromised (de-saturating, cyanotic, sternal/intercostal recessions, increased/decreased respiratory rate).
- Call the appropriate teams early including the on-call anaesthetist, ENT registrar/consultant (+/- paediatricians). If the patient is on a ward and you are concerned, put out a crash call.
- Apply high flow oxygen. Use Heliox if available.
- Give nebulised adrenaline –1ml of 1 in 1000 adrenaline diluted to 5mls with 0.9% saline. This can be repeated as necessary.
- Gain IV access, blood gases and give IV dexamethasone (adults 8mg, children 150 micrograms/kg). Do not attempt without anaesthetic/senior help if this is making the patient more distressed impacting the airway.
- Ensure the emergency airway trolley including cricothyroidotomy kit and a flexible nasendoscope are available. If the patient is stable and you are competent at using scopes, perform flexible nasendoscopy. If not, have the equipment ready. The anaesthetist should also be present to visualise and assess the airway to see if intubation is appropriate and or possible.
- If the patient is stable take a history and complete your examination to try and ascertain the cause and treat as appropriate with senior help.

Figure 28. *Initial Management of Stridor*

Post-tonsillectomy bleeds

Post-tonsillectomy bleeds can be life threatening, especially in small children. These bleeds may be primary (in the first 24 hours post-operatively) or secondary (later than 24 hours). Adult patients will report spitting out or swallowing blood, but be aware that in children presentation may be subtler with just vomiting, or excessive swallowing and volumes may therefore be underestimated.

All patients should be seen urgently and Seniors informed early. Perform an ABCD assessment ensuring patients are sat up with a bowl to spit into, have IV access and bloods have been taken (FBC, Clotting, Group & Save).

Further Management:

- Bleeding spontaneously stopped/slow ooze:
  These patients still require admission for observation, as a small bleed may precede a larger bleed. Examine the oropharynx to localise possible bleeding points or clots in the tonsillar fossae. Make the patient NBM initially until discussed with a Senior. Start hydrogen peroxide gargles, analgesia and for secondary haemorrhages, broad spectrum IV antibiotics.
- Bleeding ongoing
  These patients should be looked after in resus and the on-call anaesthetist, an ENT Senior and theatres should be contacted. Resuscitate the patient with fluids and blood products as appropriate and give IV tranexamic acid. Use forceps to apply gauze, or a tonsil swab soaked in 1 in 10,000 adrenaline to the bleeding tonsillar fossa. In heavy bleeds, the priority is organising the patient for arrest of haemorrhage in theatre. In children with ongoing bleeds consider involving the paediatric team and remember they have smaller circulating blood volumes therefore require prompt resuscitation.

Tracheostomies/laryngectomies

Nursing staff usually carry out the regular ward care of tracheostomies, but in the case of an emergency it is important that you are familiar with the emergency tracheostomy and laryngectomy algorithms produced by the National Tracheostomy Safety Project (National Tracheostomy Safety Project 2012). Tracheostomy inner tubes can easily become blocked with secretions if not cleaned regularly, so always ensure suction is available and remove the inner tube if any concern about the airway. Call for anaesthetic and Senior ENT help if suction or inner tube changes do not help and follow the emergency algorithm.

Patients will usually have a sign at their bedside indicating what type of airway they have and a bag with equipment. It is important to remember that patients with a laryngectomy do not have a patent airway via the mouth.

Post-thyroidectomy Haemorrhage

If called to recovery or the ward to attend a patient post-thyroidectomy, with any signs of respiratory difficulty or distress, attend immediately.

Post-operative neck haematomas whilst rare, are a potentially life-threatening cause of airway obstruction. Early diagnosis and immediate management are imperative. Other warning signs may include increasing neck pain, swelling and pressure sensation, dysphagia and increased blood in the neck drain (Bononi et al. 2010, 1173-1177).

If a haematoma is suspected, skin sutures and deeper sutures should be immediately removed followed by suction of the haematoma at the bedside. An ENT Senior and the on-call anaesthetist should be contacted but do not wait for them to open the wound. The obstruction may not be eased by this if laryngopharyngeal oedema has developed secondary to impairment of venous and lymphatic drainage. Urgent intubation or cricothyroidotomy may be required.

References

Ambrus P, Eavey R, Baker A, Wilson W and Kelly J. Management of Nasal Septal Abscess. *Laryngoscope*, Vol. 91, No. 4, 1981, pp. 575-582

Bartlett A, Williams R, Hilton M. Splenic rupture in infectious mononucleosis: a systematic review of published case reports. Injury. 2016 Mar 1;47(3):531-8

British Medical Journal Best Practice. 2017. "Bell's Palsy." Last Reviewed March 2019. https://newbp.bmj.com/topics/en-gb/118

Bononi M, Bonapasta SA, Vari A, Scarpini M, De Cesare A, Miccini M, Meucci M, Tocchi A. Incidence and circumstances of cervical hematoma complicating thyroidectomy and its relationship to postoperative vomiting. Head & neck. 2010 Sep;32(9):1173-7

British Soceity of Audiology. 2016. "Recommended Procedure: Rinne and Weber Tuning Fork Tests." Updated September 2016. https://www.thebsa.org.uk/wp-content/uploads/1987/04/Recommended-Procedure-Tuning-Forks-2016.pdf

Canty PA, Berkowitz RG. Hematoma and abscess of the nasal septum in children. *Arch Otolaryngol Head Neck Surg* [Internet]. 1996 Dec [cited 2016 Oct 2];122(12):1373–6

D.J Premachandra, D. MrRae, Severe tissue destruction in the ear caused by alkaline button batteries, *Postgrad Med J* (1990) 66:52-53

De Seta D, Mancini P, Minni A, Prosperini L, De Seta E, Attanasio G, Covelli E, De Carlo A, Filipo R. Bell's palsy: symptoms preceding and accompanying the facial paresis. The Scientific World Journal. 2014.

Heiden C, Porzsolt F, Biesinger E, Höing R. Spontaneous remission of sudden deafness. Hno. 2000 Aug;48(8):621-3.

J. Phillips. Evidence review and ENT-UK consensus report for the use of aminoglycoside-containing ear drops in the presence of an open middle ear. *Clin Otolaryngol.* 2007 Oct;32(5):330-6.

Ketcham AS, Han JK (2010). Complications and management of septoplasty. *Otolaryngol Clin North* Am 43: 897-904

Lee, Jong Dae, Byung Don Lee, and Sun Chul Hwang. Vestibular Schwannoma in Patients with Sudden Sensorineural Hearing Loss. *Skull Base*. 2011 Mar; 21(2): 75–78.

Lue AJ, Fang WD, Manolidis S. Use of plain radiography and computed tomography to identify fish bone foreign bodies. Otolaryngology-Head and Neck Surgery. 2000 Oct 1;123(4):435-8

National Tracheostomy Project. 2012. "Emergency Tracheostomy Algorithm" and "Emergency Laryngectomy Algorithm". Last Reviewed 2016. http://www.tracheostomy.org.uk/storage/files/Patent%20Airway%20Algorithm.pdf

NHS Quality Improvement Scotland. 2010. "Scottish Intercollegiate Guidelines Network: Management of sore throat and indications for tonsillectomy. A National Clinical Guideline" (guideline 117). https://www.sign.ac.uk/assets/sign117.pdf

Peitersen E. The natural History of Bell Palsy. Am J Otol. 1982;4: 107-111

Purohit N, Ray S, Wilson T, Chawla OP (2008). The 'Parents Kiss': an effective way to remove paediatric nasal foreign bodies. *Ann R Coll Surg Engl* 90:420-22

Tysome J, Kanegaonkar R. 2012. ENT *An Introduction And Practical Guide*. CRC Press

Warner G et al. 2009. *Otolaryngology and Head and Neck Surgery*. Oxford University Press

Weinaug P. Spontaneous remission in sudden deafness. HNP 1984;32:346-51

CHAPTER 3

GENERAL SURGERY

SIMON MCCLUNEY & CHRISTOS KONTOVOUNISIOS

Abstract
Section 1 – Appendicitis
Section 2 – Bowel Obstruction
Small bowel obstruction
Large bowel obstruction
Section 3 – Biliary Pathology
Simple biliary pathology
Complex biliary pathology
Section 4 – Pancreatitis
Section 5 – Diverticulitis
Section 6 – Herniae
Section 7 – Abscesses
Section 8 – Perianal Disease
Haemorrhoids
Perianal fissure
Perianal fistulas
Pilonidal disease
Section 9 – Bariatric Emergencies
Section 10 – Abdominal Wound Dehiscence
Section 11 – Enterocutaneous fistula
Section 12 – Perforation
Upper GI perforation
Lower GI perforation
Section 13 – High ileostomy output
Conclusion

Abstract

General surgery is the largest surgical speciality and covered extensively in undergraduate training. Whilst it can be argued that general surgery is becoming more subspecialised, this does not apply to emergency on-call shifts. General surgery presenting complaints can be life threatening if not identified and managed correctly and it is vital that junior doctors are aware of how to manage these patients safely and when to ask for Senior help. However, alongside this, there are several conditions that are only briefly covered in undergraduate training but are encountered whilst on-call and can be challenging for the inexperienced junior doctor.

This chapter covers all key general surgical conditions including appendicitis, biliary tree pathologies, bowel obstruction, hernias and bariatric emergencies. It also looks at common, but generally less serious, conditions including perianal abscesses, perianal fissures, haemorrhoids, PR bleeding and pilonidal disease.

The chapter provides the reader with an easy to follow guide to facilitate safe decision making with confidence whilst providing emergency on-call cover.

Section 1: Appendicitis

Acute appendicitis is one of the most common causes of an acute abdomen, and one of the differential diagnoses that is most often referred to surgical SHOs, with male and female lifetime incidence of 8% and 6% respectively (Addiss, Shaffe, Fowler, Taux 1990, 910). Often, patients with lower central and right sided abdominal pain will be referred to general surgery as suspected appendicitis, even if other differentials are more likely. It is therefore imperative that as the SHO, you are able to differentiate between the pertinent diagnoses, based on a comprehensive history and examination.

History and examination

Classic presenting complaint: Central abdominal pain, later radiating to right hand side, with anorexia and nausea or vomiting.

However, the early symptoms can be subtle, and non-specific symptoms include:

- Indigestion
- Change in bowel habit
- Malaise

Moreover, the chronicity of the pain can help us in the differential. For example, appendicitis is much more likely to produce a grumbling pain with increasing intensity over the course of hours to days, with gradual onset, whereas a right sided ovarian torsion is more likely to give immediate, severe pain. Patients with appendicitis often present with a low-grade pyrexia, with high fevers more common in advanced disease, such as perforation.

Although the appendix base is fixed to the caecum, the location of the appendix tip can vary greatly with different corresponding symptoms:

- Anterior: classical localised peritonism in the right iliac fossa.
- Retrocaecal: This can lead to generalised abdominal pain, or even right lumbar/upper quadrant pain, creating a diagnostic dilemma.
- Pelvic appendix: This can lead to suprapubic tenderness, or urinary symptoms.

Top differential diagnoses to consider (not inclusive): Gastroenteritis, mesenteric adenitis, Crohn's disease, diverticulitis, Meckel's diverticulitis, gynaecological pathology such as pelvic inflammatory disease, cyst rupture, mittelschmerz, ovarian torsion, ectopic pregnancy, tubo-ovarian abscess and urological conditions, such as renal colic, epididymitis and testicular torsion.

Investigations

White cell count (WCC) and C-reactive protein (CRP) play a role. There is conflicting evidence regarding WCC and CRP in acute appendicitis, however, it is established that raised WCC and CRP have been associated with more complicated disease (Sengupta, Bax, Paterson-Brown 2009, 113-115). Perhaps the most commonly used scoring system is the **Alvarado score** (Alvarado 1986, 557-564) (Table 1), which has been validated in acute appendicitis. It is perhaps most useful as a "rule out" tool, with those with a score <5 unlikely to have appendicitis (Ohle, O'Reilly, O'Brien, Fahey et al. 2011, 139). All patients should also have blood cultures if pyrexial, urinalysis including a pregnancy test and a group and save/screen if the index of suspicion is high.

Symptoms/Sign/Test	Score
Migration of Pain	1
Anorexia	1
Nausea/Vomiting	1
Tenderness in the right iliac fossa	2
Rebound tenderness	1
Raised temperature (≥37.3)	1
Leucocyte count ≥10x10^9/L	2
Differential white cell count with neutrophils ≥75%	1
Total	10

Table 1. *The Alvarado Score (Alvarado 1986)*

In young males with a classical history, imaging is typically unnecessary and often unhelpful. However, if the history is suggestive of alternative pathology, such as inflammatory bowel disease, imaging should be considered. In those over 40 years old, cross-sectional imaging should be considered due to the possibility of other potential diagnoses, such as a right sided malignancy or diverticulitis. Females will often undergo a trans-abdominal +/- trans-vaginal ultrasound scan if a gynaecological pathology is suspected. The diagnosis can be difficult in pregnant women, due to displacement of the appendix by the expanding uterus, and the leucocytosis associated with pregnancy. Thus, MRI is the gold standard in such patients and should be considered, however, not at the risk of delaying treatment. In such complex patients, early Senior input should be sought.

Management

Patients are typically resuscitated with intravenous fluids, and if likely for surgery, are fasted as appropriate. In septic patients, antibiotics should be started whilst investigations are underway. However, in those with equipoise and no signs of sepsis, antibiotics may mask the symptoms of a progressing early appendicitis. In such patients, antibiotics may be temporarily withheld, and serial clinical examination performed until a more definitive diagnosis can be made. It is, however, imperative that such patients are closely monitored. Senior support should be sought in this scenario.

The current standard treatment for acute appendicitis is surgery, however, in those patients with a suspected appendix mass, long-term antibiotics may be commenced and an interval appendicectomy performed in the outpatient setting, at least 8 weeks after the original pathology. In patients with a pelvic or intra-abdominal abscess, percutaneous or transrectal image guided drainage can be performed to reduce the burden of sepsis.

There is evidence to suggest that conservative management has at least equivalent outcomes to surgery in uncomplicated appendicitis, however, the caveat is that patients have a 30% chance of developing repeat appendicitis within 1 year, and a 1/10 chance of needing a rescue appendicectomy at the index presentation (Vons, Barry, Maitre, Pautrat et al. 2011, 1573). In the United Kingdom, surgical intervention is the current standard of care, but conservative management considered for patients who are averse to having surgery. Laparoscopic appendicectomy is performed in most patients, with open appendicectomy reserved primarily for paediatric patients. In paediatric surgical centres, however, laparoscopic appendicectomy is the standard of care for most patients. The RIFT national audit in 2017, demonstrated an initial laparoscopic approach of 94% in females, compared to 91% in males. This is in comparison to a rate of 66% in 2012 (RIFT Study Group 2018, 55).

Section 2: Bowel Obstruction

Surgical SHOs are often referred patients with suspected bowel obstruction. Such patients should be reviewed expediently to delineate the underlying pathology and begin early investigation and management. **Small bowel obstruction is more common than large bowel obstruction**, with the small bowel involved in intestinal obstruction in approximately 80% of cases (Drożdż, Budzyński 2012, 175-180)

Small bowel obstruction

The three most common causes of small bowel obstruction are:

- Adhesions
- Herniae
- Malignancy

Other, rarer, causes include strictures secondary to inflammatory bowel pathology, volvulus, intussusception, gallstones and foreign bodies.

Common presenting symptoms:

- Nausea ± vomiting
- Cramping abdominal pain
- Obstipation

In some patients, this may be abrupt and constant, whilst in others it may be intermittent and resolve, only to recur later. Moreover, some patients may describe a longer history of sub-acute obstruction, which has progressed to acute obstruction. Such patients should have a thorough clerking, including a systematic abdominal examination including palpation for any herniae, which can occasionally be missed by the referring doctor. Patients should have a digital rectal examination for any rectal mass or impaction, whilst the presence of blood could indicate either a cause for the obstruction, such as malignancy, or a complication such as ischaemia.

Investigations

These patients should be investigated with:

- Bloods: full blood count, urea and electrolytes, C-reactive protein and an arterial blood gas with a lactate. A normal lactate, however, should not be used as reassurance that the bowel is healthy – patients can have a small amount of ischaemic bowel and still have a normal lactate.
- Imaging:
    - Plain abdominal and erect chest radiographs, to quickly determine if obstruction is present, along with any free intra-abdominal air. Classical features are distended small bowel loops with air-fluid levels, however, one must be careful in patients with equivocal radiographs, as even those with a "gasless abdomen" on X-ray can have complete small bowel obstruction with the dilated loops full of fluid. Additionally, those with a proximal obstruction, e.g. proximal jejunum, may have minimal dilated loops on plain radiographs (Figure 1a).

    - If there is diagnostic uncertainty, or the site and cause of obstruction is unknown, patients should proceed to abdominal and pelvic CT scan. This is much more useful for determining the site and degree of obstruction. Bowel obstruction can be partial or complete, whilst a closed loop obstruction occurs when there are 2 points of obstruction with a subsequent segment of bowel with no inlet or outlet. Such patients are at high risk of perforation (Figure 1b).

Figure 1: *A) Abdominal radiograph demonstrating small bowel obstruction (*Heilman 1a); *B) Axial image of a computerised tomography scan demonstrating small bowel obstruction. The red arrow indicates the air/fluid level typical of bowel obstruction (*Heilman 1b).
See colour centrefold for this image.

Management

The treatment of small bowel obstruction, either surgical or conservative management, often depends on the aetiology. Broadly speaking, in a clinically well patient with partial obstruction due to suspected adhesions, non-operative management may be instigated.

The widely used term "drip and suck" refers to patients receiving intravenous fluids (drip) and intestinal decompression via a naso-gastric tube (suck). The NG tube should be a large bore Ryle's tube, for example, 14-20Fr dependent on the size of the patient, whilst it should be on free drainage (i.e. bowel contents will freely drain into the bag), with 2-4 hourly aspirates. Such patients may also be given a water-soluble contrast agent, such as Gastrografin, which can help to stimulate intestinal peristalsis. **This can be used in partial obstruction, but not in complete or closed loop obstruction as it could cause a perforation**. Gastrografin is widely used in the UK to diagnose and/or treat suspected adhesional obstruction, however, the evidence for its benefits remains conflicting. Typically, most centres will have a guideline in place for its dosing, or this can be discussed with Seniors/pharmacy and the radiologist who will be reporting the X-ray. If the patient has suspected bowel obstruction, they will almost always have a NG tube. In this case, the gastrograffin can be introduced via the NG tube, and the NG should be spigotted (i.e. temporarily blocked), so that it does not reflux into the drainage bag.

Indications for surgical intervention include complete obstruction, closed loop obstruction, evidence of peritonitis suggesting ischaemia, perforation or necrosis and failure of non-operative management. For patients who are managed conservatively, they should have serial examination to ensure they are not developing complications, and if the symptoms are not settling by 48 hours, considered for surgical intervention. Resolution is suggested by reduced distension, reduced nasogastric tube output and passage of flatus and/or stool. **Irreducible herniae causing small bowel obstruction should be surgically managed**. In suspected malignancy, the decision should be made based upon the patient's clinical status, the nature of the suspected tumour, their co-morbidities and the overall goal of treatment.

Large bowel obstruction

Large bowel obstruction often has a more sinister pathology and is the presenting symptom in approximately 30% of colorectal cancer (Buechter, Boustany, Caillouette, Cohn 1988, 163-168). The most common benign pathology is volvulus, such as sigmoid volvulus, whilst other aetiologies include adhesions, repeated diverticular disease, herniae, ischaemic colitis and inflammatory bowel disease. Large bowel obstruction is a surgical emergency, and the surgical mantra of: "Do not let the sun set on a bowel obstruction", is highly relevant. Seek Senior advice and input early for these patients.

Differential diagnoses include: small bowel obstruction, toxic megacolon, ileus – where the entire intestinal tract will be distended, and Ogilvie's syndrome, where imaging fails to identify a mechanical cause or transition point. Like small bowel obstruction, these patients can present acutely or with chronic symptoms, and thus, the history is critical in helping to elucidate the underlying pathology.

Investigations

Such patients should have similar laboratory studies, in addition to a carcinoembryonic antigen (CEA) level, which is typically raised in malignancy. Again, patients should have plain radiography and likely proceed to CT scanning. Plain films are useful and can have characteristic findings in some conditions, such as sigmoid volvulus, with the coffee bean sign demonstrated in Figure 2 below.

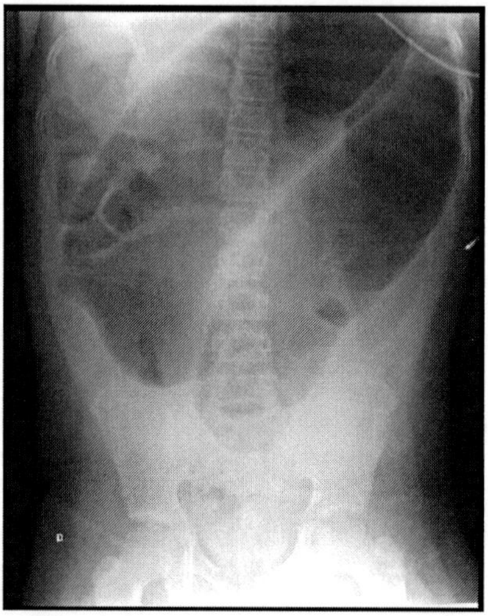

Figure 2: *Abdominal radiograph demonstrating sigmoid volvulus with the characteristic coffee bean sign Please not this is Xray is of a child but the. (Wikipedia 2019)*

Management

As opposed to small bowel obstruction, **most large bowel obstructions require surgical intervention**. For malignancy, this mandates a bowel resection, or for patients felt unsuitable for surgery, colonic stenting or surgical diversion is a suitable alternative. Patients with a sigmoid volvulus may initially be managed with flatus tube insertion after seeking Senior support, with an inpatient flexible sigmoidoscopy to adequately decompress the colon and visualise the affected area. In patients with recurrent sigmoid volvulus, a sigmoid colectomy should be considered.

Section 3: Biliary Pathology

Gallstones are very common in Western world; however, the majority of patients are asymptomatic. Symptomatic patients can be broadly classified into 4 groups:

- Simple biliary pathology:
    - Symptomatic gallstone disease (biliary colic)

- Complex biliary pathology:
    - o Acute cholecystitis
    - o Gallstone pancreatitis
    - o Pyrexia & jaundice due to gallstone disease

Simple biliary pathology

The most common symptomatic pathology is biliary colic. This is characterised by a dull pain in the right upper quadrant with intermittent bouts of increased intensity. It may radiate to the back and be associated with nausea and vomiting. Blood tests should be normal in these patients, and the abdominal examination should be relatively unremarkable. In patients with known gallstones with suspected biliary colic, they can be managed as an outpatient unless they require admission for strong analgesia. In patients with no prior history, they should have a transabdominal ultrasound scan during this presentation, or this can be arranged expediently in centres that have a surgical "hot" clinic. As an outpatient, the patients should be advised to have a low-fat diet.

Such patients should have a laparoscopic cholecystectomy ideally within 6 weeks of initial presentation. Inpatients with intractable pain should be managed as acute cholecystitis, and have a laparoscopic cholecystectomy (LC) on their index admission.

Complex biliary pathology

In patients with symptoms persisting for 24 hours, peritonism in the right upper quadrant, abnormal blood tests (white cell count, liver function tests) or pyrexia, a diagnosis of cholecystitis should be considered. These patients should be admitted, commenced on antibiotics and intravenous fluids, and an ultrasound scan arranged for the following day. If peritonism is present, an erect chest radiograph should be considered to rule out a perforated viscus.

Patients with acute cholecystitis should have a Laparoscopic Cholecystectomy (LC) within 72 hours as per NICE guidelines, however, this should be done by a surgeon with a sub-specialism in upper GI surgery, or transferred to an alternative centre (National Institute for Health and Care Excellence, CG188). There is, however, a vast difference in the uptake of this recommendation across the country, and the previous treatment choice of a course of antibiotics followed by a "cold"/outpatient cholecystectomy is still encountered in a lot of hospitals.

Patients who are unfit for surgery can potentially be treated with a percutaneous cholecystostomy placed by interventional radiology. This allows for drainage of the infection. In patients with grossly deranged liver function tests, suggestive of an obstructive picture, common bile duct calculi (choledocholithiasis) should be considered. These patients may require further biliary imaging, such as an MRCP, and an ERCP for definitive diagnosis and management. Most centres have guidelines relating to the management of acute gallstone pathology and the various options available (such as LC with on-table cholangiogram +/- bile duct exploration, or LC with post-operative ERCP) dependent on the degree of suspicion for CBD stones.

In patients with suspected cholangitis, the **sepsis protocol** should be followed, senior support sought and an ERCP may be required as an emergency to clear the biliary tree. In patients with mild to moderate disease, an ERCP can be performed within 24-48 hours, however, in those with severe cholangitis, it should be performed within 24 hours. This can be difficult depending on local resources, and in some cases, may require transfer to a tertiary centre for urgent ERCP. Where ERCP is not available or not possible due to anatomy, such as a Roux-En-Y anastomosis, percutaneous drainage is an acceptable alternative. Percutaneous transhepatic cholangiography allows placement of a biliary drain to drain the sepsis. LC is recommended after ERCP for jaundice or cholangitis secondary to CBD stones. After cholangitis, this can be very technically challenging and should be done by a HPB surgeon.

Section 4: Pancreatitis

Epigastric pain is a common complaint referred to general surgery. The differentials include:

- Peptic ulcer disease
- Gallstone disease
- Perforation
- Mesenteric ischaemia
- Bowel obstruction
- Non-general surgery causes such as acute coronary syndrome and ruptured AAA

The most common causes of pancreatitis are gallstones and alcohol, however, there are many other well-established causes. Pancreatitis can be diagnosed based upon meeting 2 of 3 criteria:

- Classical symptomatic presentation
- Amylase or lipase greater than 3 times the normal limit
- Radiological findings suggestive of acute pancreatitis based on CT or MRI

Pancreatitis can be classified into mild (no evidence of organ failure), moderately severe (transient organ failure less than 48 hours) and severe (persistent organ failure). There are multiple scoring systems based on biochemical and radiological criteria, however, in the UK, the most commonly used is the Glasgow-Imrie score. The mnemonic for remembering this is PANCREAS, (Table 2). This is an 8-point scale and if the score is 3 or greater, there is a high chance of severe pancreatitis. **Such patients should have critical care input**. 20% of patients have moderately severe or severe pancreatitis, however, the remaining 80% should recover within 5 days.

Test Result	Score
PaO2 <8kPa	1
Age >55 years	1
WBC >15 x10^9/L (**N**eutrophils)	1
Serum **C**alcium <2mmol/L	1
Serum Urea >16mmol/L (**R**enal)	1
LDH >600IU/L (**E**nzymes)	1
Serum **A**lbumin <32g/L	1
Blood glucose >10mmol/L (**S**ugar)	1

Table 2. *Glasglow Acute Pancreatitis Severity Score (Blamey, Imrie, O'Neill 1984, 1340-1346)*

Approximately 15% of patients will have pancreatic necrosis, and other local complications include peri-pancreatic collections, portal venous system thrombosis and pseudocysts, shown in Figure 4.

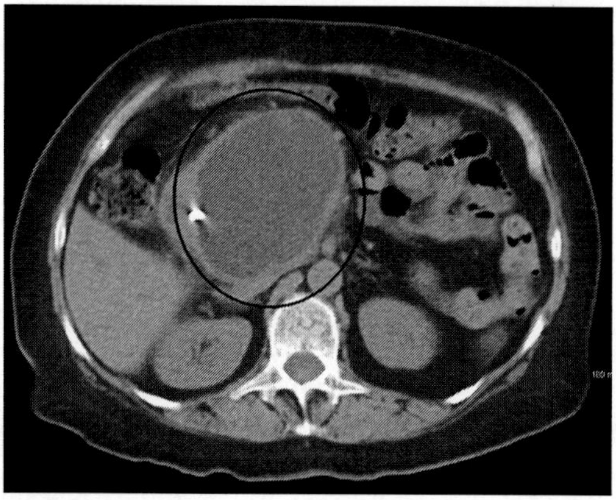

Figure 3: *Axial slice of a computerised tomography scan demonstrating a large pancreatic pseudocyst with compression with the left renal vessels (Heilman 1e).*

Investigations

All patients should have a full blood count, U&Es, LFTs, CRP and an erect chest radiograph to exclude free air. Either amylase or lipase is used to aid in the diagnosis; amylase is more commonly used but lipase is gaining popularity. If the diagnosis is uncertain, a CT scan should be performed. A pregnancy test should be sought in females of a child bearing age. Patients with an unknown aetiology should have a transabdominal ultrasound scan. If this is negative, a lipid profile can be ordered to check for hypertriglyceridaemia. In middle-aged and elderly patients with severe epigastric pain radiating to the back, one must consider the possibility of a ruptured/leaking abdominal aortic aneurysm.

Management

Patients should be commenced on aggressive fluid resuscitation, **5-10ml/kg/hour** is a reasonable starting point, providing there are no contraindications based on co-morbidities. This should be goal directed based on heart rate, blood pressure and urine output. Aggressive resuscitation should be limited to the first 24-48 hours, as after this, it is associated with increased risk of intubation and abdominal compartment syndrome (Vege, Whitcomb, Grover 2018).

Patients should have liberal analgesia, which may mandate patient controlled opioid analgesia. Oral feeding can be slowly commenced from 24 hours in the absence of nausea, vomiting and ileus. A systematic review indicated no adverse effects of early instigation of enteral feeding (<48 hours) (Vaughn, Shuster, Rogers, Mann et al. 2017, 883-892). There is no role for prophylactic antibiotics, however, up to 20% of patients will develop an extra-pancreatic infection which clinicians should be mindful of (Besselink, van Santvoort, Boermeester, Nieuwenhuijs et al., 2009, 267-73). Patients with moderately severe or severe pancreatitis, or no clinical improvement after 72 hours should undergo a repeat CT scan to assess for complications. Patients with complications or persistent organ failure should be transferred to an HPB centre.

In patients with proven mild gallstone pancreatitis, they should ideally have an LC on the index admission, or within 2-weeks as an outpatient. If they are unfit for surgery, they should have an ERCP with sphincterotomy as a preventative measure and a subsequent LC. Patients with severe pancreatitis should be managed as appropriate, and when recovered, can have an LC as an outpatient.

Section 5: Diverticulitis

Diverticulitis is a common referral to the acute surgical take. It is defined as a micro or macro perforation of a diverticulum. It is most commonly present in the sigmoid colon, and therefore most patients will present with left sided abdominal pain. They may also have fever, nausea and change in bowel habit. Urinary symptoms may occur due to bladder irritation.

It can be broadly categorised into uncomplicated and complicated. Complicated diverticulitis is associated with an abscess (Hinchey classification grades 1-4), obstruction, perforation or fistula. It is common in older populations, with a mean age of 63 years. In patients with no known history of diverticular disease, or an atypical history, a CT scan should be obtained to ensure there is no other pathology, such as a malignancy.

This is in addition to the standard laboratory tests outlined previously, and these patients will typically have a leucocytosis and raised CRP.

Management

Patients with a known history of diverticular disease, who are clinically well with no pyrexia and reassuring blood tests, can be managed with outpatient antibiotics. However, with fever and raised inflammatory markers patients should be admitted and commenced on intravenous antibiotics and fluids. Patients with no prior history should also be admitted for investigations and management. If there is a concern for complicated diverticulitis, such as sepsis or localised peritonism, patients should undergo a CT scan. Although there is no evidence for dietary restriction in uncomplicated diverticulitis, the standard of practice in most hospitals is for patients to be progressed from nil by mouth, to a liquid and then solid diet as their symptoms resolve (Vennix, Morton, Hahnloser, Lange et al. 2014, 866-78).

For patients with a free perforation, either demonstrated on imaging or on clinical examination, surgical intervention is mandated. Patients with abscesses can potentially be managed with antibiotics and/or percutaneous drainage, however, failure of medical management is an indication for surgical intervention. Additionally, those with obstruction should also undergo surgical resection. In uncomplicated disease, patients who do not improve after 2-3 days of conservative management, should be re-imaged to assess for complications and the potential need for surgery.

Patients can be discharged once their vital signs have normalised, their abdominal pain has abated and leucocytosis resolved. After the complete resolution of symptoms (typically 6-8 weeks), patients should have a full colonoscopy to assess the extent of their disease and to exclude a malignancy.

Section 6: Herniae

Herniae are a very common source of referrals for surgical SHOs, and for those with little experience, they can be challenging in their assessment and management. Inguinal herniae are the most common presentation to the emergency department, however, femoral herniae are responsible for more complications. Herniae may present in a variety of ways, with some patients only experiencing mild discomfort, through to those with strangulated herniae and bowel obstruction.

Examination

Examination is key, and can prove challenging for junior clinicians. This is especially true for inguinal herniae. All patients should be examined lying and standing, with the groin area completely exposed. Firstly, all herniae should be assessed for reducibility. If a hernia is completely reducible with minimal discomfort, there is typically no urgent clinical concern. If a hernia is irreducible, and especially if it is tender, this is more concerning. Large inguino-scrotal herniae may immediately prolapse after reduction, but as long as reduction is possible with minimal discomfort and no worrisome signs or symptoms, an emergency repair is typically unnecessary. One can assess whether an inguinal hernia is likely to be direct or indirect based on examination findings. If the hernia is successfully reduced, and direct pressure is placed over the deep inguinal ring, on coughing, an indirect hernia should not recur, whereas a direct hernia is more likely to recur. This is not an exact science but can give a reasonable estimate.

Femoral herniae are more likely to become irreducible or "stuck", as opposed to inguinal herniae. An incisional hernia is any hernia over the location of a previous surgical incision. A ventral hernia refers to any hernia occurring on the anterior abdominal wall.

Clinicians can sometimes appear to use terms such as incarceration with different meanings.

- Incarceration is the trapping of hernia contents preventing reduction, i.e. an irreducible hernia. If an irreducible hernia contains bowel, this can result in bowel obstruction (Figure 4).
- Strangulation is loss of the blood supply to the hernia contents, resulting in ischaemia and necrosis.

An innocuous hernia may be uncomfortable with discomfort on examination, however, it should not be tender. A tender hernia should be investigated thoroughly. Additionally, a patient with a strangulated hernia and bowel compromise may have a normal lactate, thus a lactate should not be used as a falsely reassuring test.

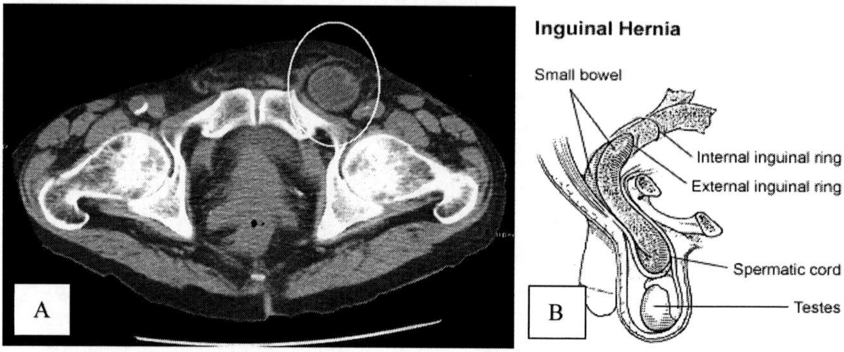

Figures 4: *A) An axial slice of a computerised tomography scan of an incarcerated left inguinal hernia containing bowel (*Heilman 1c). *B) A schematic demonstrating inguinal herniae anatomy (NIHR);*

Investigation

Routine blood tests should be performed, especially if an operative repair is likely. A blood lactate should be taken from each patient, however, as mentioned previously, should not be reassuring if normal with a high clinical suspicion of strangulation. Imaging is not typically required but can be used for occult herniae and when the diagnosis is uncertain. In such patients with suspected simple groin/abdominal wall herniae, ultrasonography should suffice. In patients with complex abdominal wall herniae, or groin/abdominal wall herniae with possible intra-abdominal complications, computed tomography is the test of choice.

Management

Patients with a strangulation or associated bowel obstruction should undergo urgent surgery within four to six hours of the onset of symptoms. Those with an incarcerated hernia but no evidence of strangulation (skin changes, peritonism), should be offered an urgent repair. Patients can also undergo an attempt at manual reduction, and if successful, should be re-assessed in the following days to exclude a recurrent incarceration and arrange for elective repair.

In patients with femoral herniae, early elective repair is recommended due to the high risk of complications. For those with a long-standing femoral hernia who are not keen for intervention, watchful waiting can be considered.

Section 7: Abscesses

General surgeons are generally responsible for abscesses on: abdomen, trunk, axilla, groin, scalp and posterior neck triangle. Abscess management is primarily incision and drainage. Local policies are often in place for patients to return the following morning, or a similar arrangement, for patients to have an expedited operation. The use of antibiotics post-operatively depends on the clinician, however, as a rule of thumb, patients with the following criteria should complete a course of antibiotics:

- Abscess >2cm
- Multiple abscesses
- Extensive cellulitis
- Fever
- Inadequate response to incision and drainage.

Generally speaking, a significant number of abscess drainages can be done under local anaesthetic in the emergency department, and the A&E team may deal with small, uncomplicated abscesses. Considerations include the size of the abscess, systemic infection and patient preference. Perianal abscesses should always be drained under general anaesthesia due to pain and also as one must perform a thorough EUA to check for a fistula. In most cases, axillary abscesses and pilonidal abscesses also require general anaesthesia due to pain.

Otherwise simple local anaesthetic can be used, either as an injection, or with a numbing spray, such as ethyl chloride, which is usually present in emergency departments. Breast abscesses are typically managed conservatively with antibiotics +/- ultrasound guided aspiration in the first instance. Patients who do not respond, or are systemically unwell, will proceed to surgical intervention, usually performed by a specialist breast surgeon.

Section 8: Perianal Disease

Haemorrhoids

Haemorrhoids are classified in relation to the dentate line, with those lying proximally at/above the dentate line, known as internal haemorrhoids, and those below, as external haemorrhoids (Figure 5). External haemorrhoids are more likely to be painful, due to somatic innervation below the dentate line. Internal haemorrhoids have 4 classifications:

- Grade 1 – bulge without prolapse
- Grade 2 – prolapse with spontaneous reduction
- Grade 3 – prolapse beyond the dentate line requiring manual reduction
- Grade 4 – prolapsed haemorrhoids that cannot be reduced

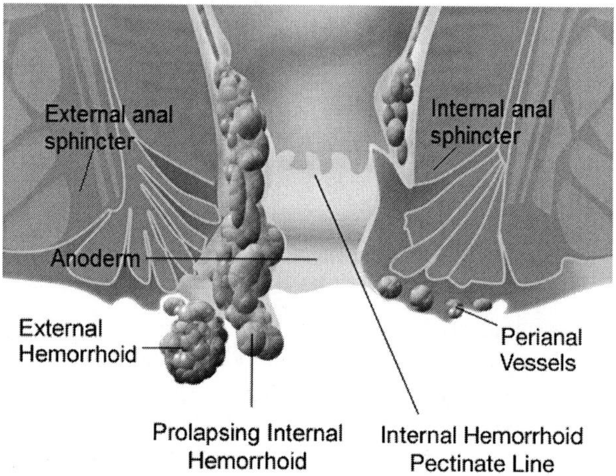

Figure 5*: Internal and external haemorrhoids (*Häggström).

The most common presentation to A&E is due to bleeding. If the patient is stable with a normal haemoglobin and on examination the bleeding is obviously due to haemorrhoids, i.e. bleeding on contact, and there is no suspicion of proximal GI bleeding, such patients can be discharged with appropriate outpatient follow up. It is very rare for surgical intervention to be required for haemorrhoidal bleeding. This is usually limited to patients with coagulopathy.

Haemorrhoids presenting with pain, again, should not require inpatient admission. Such patients should be advised to use topical anaesthetic creams/gels, such as hydrocortisone/lidocaine preparations and regular Sitz bathes. Patients with thrombosed external haemorrhoids again should not require admission and are managed as above, however, some individual clinicians may perform surgical management if analgesia fails. Thrombosed external haemorrhoids can similarly be managed with topical applications, and a cold flannel or ice packs can be applied to the area to reduce discomfort and swelling. Such patients are often referred by community doctors, and telephone advice is typically all that is required, avoiding a hospital attendance.

Perianal Fissure

Perianal fissures are a common cause of acute perianal pain and bleeding. The pain is usually associated with defaecation, and the fissure can be identified on examination. Patients are usually managed with Sitz baths, topical analgesics and topical nifedipine or nitroglycerin to reduce anal sphincter pressure, aid healing and reduce pain. Similarly, such patients should not require admission. Surgical intervention is generally only performed in those with chronic fissures unresponsive to medical management, and not as an emergency.

Perianal Fistula

Perianal fistulas, or fistulas-in-ano, are the result of a previous perianal abscess which has formed an epithelised tract connecting the anorectum to the skin. Such patients usually present with a non-healing abscess, or chronic purulent discharge. Fistulae should always be considered in patients with recurrent perianal abscesses, and such patients should have an examination under anaesthetic of the anorectum at the time of incision and drainage, with outpatient follow up, with or without MRI, to delineate the underlying anatomy. In a patient with a perianal fistula and no acute infection, they can be managed as an outpatient and seen in the surgical clinic. If there is evidence of perianal sepsis, they may require admission and work up as an inpatient.

In patients with perianal fistulae or recurrent perianal abscesses, one must be mindful of the potential for an underlying diagnoses of inflammatory bowel disease. Patients with complex perianal pathology should have senior colorectal input, as decision making and correct and timely management of these patients is imperative. The anatomy of perianal fistulae can be complicated, and the most common types are demonstrated in Figure 7.

Figure 6: *Types of perianal fistulae based on their location in relation to the anal sphincters (Mcort)*
See colour centrefold for this image.

Pilonidal Disease

Patients with pilonidal disease may present to the emergency department with pilonidal abscesses. To clarify, pilonidal disease refers to the presence of pits and sinuses within the natal cleft, but with no superadded infection. A pilonidal abscess occurs with an infection in addition to the underlying pathology. Patients with an abscess should have an incision and drainage of the abscess either under local, or more commonly, general anaesthetic. It is not possible to excise the pilonidal disease when there is active infection. These patients should be followed up in the outpatient setting, as they may require an elective pilonidal sinus excision +/- reconstruction. Similarly, patients with a new diagnosis of simple pilonidal disease should be seen in the outpatient clinic to discuss management options.

Section 9: Bariatric Emergencies

The frequency of bariatric operations is increasing in the UK. Bariatric patients are generally advised to contact their operating hospital if they are symptomatic, however, they will of course present to other emergency departments. The most common bariatric operations are:

- Roux-en-Y gastric bypass (open or laparoscopic)
- Sleeve gastrectomy
- Adjustable gastric band, shown in Figure 7

Patients presenting with abdominal symptoms with a background of previous bariatric surgery should have a very careful and thorough clinical assessment. Senior input should be sought early as even in the presence of severe pathology, their symptoms may appear innocuous. Of course, bariatric patients can also suffer from typical general surgical pathology, however, they should be investigated with additional considerations.

In a patient with significant abdominal symptoms in the early post-operative period, a patient who has undergone a gastric bypass or sleeve gastrectomy should be assumed to have an anastomotic leak until proven otherwise. Such patients should have a CT with oral and IV contrast expediently. Furthermore, bowel obstruction in the post-operative period following gastric bypass should be treated as an **internal hernia** until proven otherwise. These patients usually require urgent surgical exploration to prevent catastrophic surgical complications. Patients with abdominal complaints with an adjustable gastric band, can have the band deflated in the emergency department with a Huber needle, however, senior support should be sought regarding performing this for those inexperienced with bariatric patients.

Figure 7: *Images demonstrating A) Roux-en-Y gastric bypass (Blaus); B) adjustable gastric band (Xopusmagnumx)*
See colour centrefold for this image.

Section 10: Abdominal Wound Dehiscence

All surgical wounds are at risk of wound dehiscence. The risk is increased in patients who have undergone emergency surgery with intra-abdominal contamination. Small pockets of superficial wound dehiscence are not particularly uncommon and are not a cause for concern. They will typically be managed with packing and heal by secondary intention (i.e. spontaneously and not by surgery). However, occasionally, a patient can suffer a full abdominal dehiscence, sometimes also referred to as a burst abdomen. This is a surgical emergency and is a scary prospect for all clinicians. Such patients will have a full breakdown of the surgical wound, including the abdominal wall. They may have evisceration (protrusion) of their abdominal contents. An early warning sign of this happening is pink serous discharge from the abdominal wound.

The immediate management consists of applying a non-adhesive dressing to the area, such as simple clingfilm. These patients will need an urgent exploration and closure under general anaesthetic. They will require resuscitation and early Senior involvement from the outset.

Section 11: Enterocutaneous fistulae

An enterocutaneous fistula is a tract that develops between the gastrointestinal tract and the skin. They typically develop after intestinal surgery, but also in the setting of trauma, or in inflammatory bowel disease. Emergency surgery, sepsis and malnutrition also increase the risk of developing a fistula post-operatively.

A high output fistula is defined as >500ml of affluent in 24 hours. One must ensure that an intra-abdominal abscess/ongoing sepsis has been excluded and the management consists of careful fluid balance with adequate nutrition, wound management and reducing intestinal secretions. Thus, these patients may have complete bowel rest with total parenteral nutrition, whilst octreotide can help in high output fistulae. These patients can be extremely challenging to manage and require specialist input.

Section 12: Perforation

Perforation of an intra-abdominal viscus is an acute surgical emergency. These can generally be divided into upper GI (stomach and duodenum), or lower GI (small intestine or colonic). **Any perforation is a true acute surgical emergency, and should be managed as such.** Patients with an upper GI perforation will have a chemical peritonitis from gastric and biliary contents, whilst those with a lower GI perforation will have a faecal peritonitis.

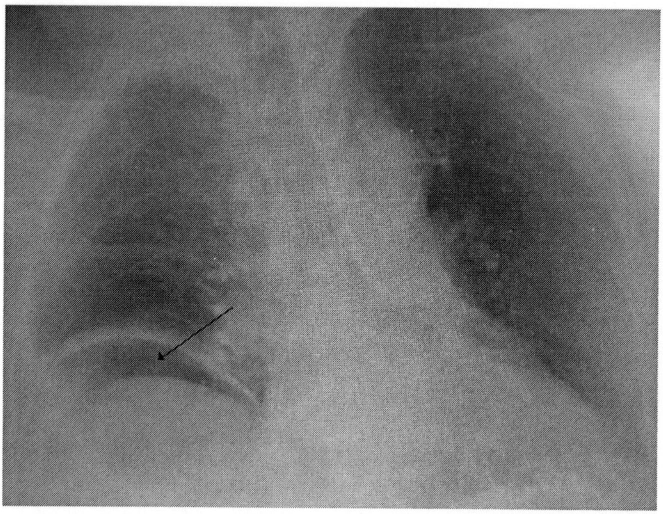

Figure 8: *Erect chest radiograph demonstrating free intra-peritoneal air under the right hemi-diaphragm (Heilman 1d)*

Perforations can present in two forms. The first is a free perforation, i.e. diffuse free intra-peritoneal air (Figure 8). These patients will be very unwell and will require surgery. The other form is a localised perforation, i.e. the perforation has occurred but has been sealed off, for example, by omentum, and formed a collection. This is more commonly encountered in the sub-acute setting, or in those with a delayed presentation. In these patients there are two options: if systemically unwell, surgery may be the preferred course, however, if they are clinically well, a conservative approach with percutaneous drainage of the abscess, for example by interventional radiology, may be adopted. All patients with perforations should have early Senior led investigation and management.

Upper GI Perforation

Upper GI, i.e. oesophago-gastric or duodenal perforations, are most commonly seen on the background of peptic ulcer disease. However, there are a plethora of other causes, such as medication, e.g. NSAIDs, ingested substances, violent retching and/or vomiting, or iatrogenic injury, e.g. during OGD or ERCP. Perforation may be on a background of chronic peptic ulcer disease; however, it occasionally may mark the first presentation of the disease. Such patients will typically have acute epigastric and/or chest pain, with symptoms of nausea and vomiting. There may be an identifiable event, such as fish-bone ingestion or prolonged vomiting, whilst classically they will want to lie or sit still, to try and reduce peritoneal irritation, and they will require strong analgesia. Elderly patients, children, or those on immunosuppressants, however, can present with minimal symptoms.

These patients should be investigated with an erect chest radiograph in Accident and Emergency, with routine bloods including full blood count, urea and electrolytes, liver function tests, amylase/lipase, C-reactive protein and an arterial lactate sample. They should have a crossmatch performed, and blood cultures if pyrexial. The sepsis pathway should be instigated, with early antibiotics, aggressive resuscitation and IV PPI therapy. Most centres will obtain a CT scan for these patients, however, if there is clinical evidence of a perforation, they may proceed straight to surgery. However, cross-sectional imaging can help with surgical planning. These patients will typically have a surgical repair with closure of the defect and an omental patch to reinforce the area. They can be approached via a traditional laparotomy, or via a laparoscopic approach.

Lower GI Perforation

Lower gastrointestinal perforations are typically due to either an obstructing mass, or diverticular disease. They will typically present with severe lower abdominal pain, and will have peritonism on examination. The presentation may be acute as above, or occasionally delayed, and such patients may present with an abdominal mass. As with upper GI perforations, they should be investigated similarly, and these patients will typically have a CT scan.

Often with faecal peritonitis, these patients will be very unwell. Surgery, unless the decision to palliate is made, is almost always mandated for such patients. The type of surgery depends on the location and type of perforation, and as opposed to upper GI perforations, these patients will typically have a resection of the affected segment, and a defunctioning proximal ostomy. A colorectal anastomosis is typically not undertaken due to the high risk of an anastomotic leak.

All patients undergoing major abdominal surgery, such as a laparotomy, should have a P-POSSUM score calculated. This is a risk prediction tool to calculate the morbidity and mortality for these patients. This should be clearly documented during the pre-operative period and discussed with the patient at the time of consent. This can also aid in the decision making as to whether surgical management is appropriate for the patient.

Section 13: High ileostomy output

High ileostomy outputs are described as greater than 1200ml of affluent over 24 hours. It is important that such patients are closely monitored and managed appropriately, with useful advice outlined below:

- Monitor for signs of dehydration and electrolyte imbalances
- Hydration replacement for volumes >1000ml/24hr with 1:1 replacement with 0.9% NaCl + 20 mmol/L KCl
- Separate solids and liquids by 30 min
- Avoid hyperosmolar beverages (ie. sweetened juices, carbonated beverages)
- Dietician input and increase intake of foods that can thicken outputs (i.e. rice, toast, bananas, cheese)
- Antidiarrheals (do not start until discussing with senior)
    - 1st line: Lomotil (max. dose 5 mg QDS)
    - 2nd line: Loperamide (max. dose 4 mg QDS)
    - 3rd line: Codeine (starting dose 30 mg QDS)
    - 4th line: Cholestyramine (starting dose 1-2 sachets daily)

Conclusion

For SHOs covering general surgery, there is a wide range of pathology. The on-calls are generally busy and the patients can be very unwell. Most SHOs will be familiar with basic aspects of general surgery from their undergraduate training and early postgraduate years. Registrars are generally based on-site, and thus should always be consulted regarding sick patients, and those that may need to go to theatre. In most centres the SHOs take the referrals, and whilst this can be a daunting prospect at first, one should always seek advice if unsure and not be afraid to ask for help.

References

A practical score for the early diagnosis of acute appendicitis. Alvarado A. Annals of Emergency Medicine. 1986 May; 15(5): 557-564

Amoxicillin plus clavulanic acid versus appendicectomy for treatment of acute uncomplicated appendicitis: an open-label, non-inferiority, randomised controlled trial. Vons C, Barry C, Maitre S, Pautrat K, L, Econte M, Costaglioli B, Karoui M al., Lancet. 2011;377(9777):1573.

Blaus, B. https://upload.wikimedia.org/wikipedia/commons/5/5c/Blausen_0776_Roux-En-Y_01.png. Creative commons license held at: https://creativecommons.org/licenses/by-sa/4.0), via Wikimedia Commons, last accessed 15/01/19

Change in mechanical bowel obstruction demographic and etiological patterns during the past century: observations from one health care institution. Drożdż W, Budzyński P. Arch Surg. 2012 Feb;147(2):175-80.

Cholelithiasis and cholecystitis. Gallstone disease: diagnosis and management (CG188). National Institute for Health and Care Excellence. https://www.nice.org.uk/guidance/cg188. Last accessed 14/03/19

Early versus delayed feeding in patients with acute pancreatitis: a systematic review. Vaughn VM, Shuster D, Rogers MA, Mann J, Conte ML, Saint S, Chopra V. Annals of internal medicine. 2017 Jun 20;166(12):883-92.

Häggström M. https://en.wikipedia.org/wiki/Hemorrhoid#/media/File:Internal_and_external_hemorrhoids.png. Creative commons licence held at: http://creativecommons.org/licenses/by-sa/3.0/, via Wikimedia Commons, last accessed 15/01/19

Heilman J, 1a. https://en.wikipedia.org/wiki/Bowel_obstruction. Creative commons licence held at: https://creativecommons.org/licenses/by-sa/3.0) from Wikimedia Commons, last accessed 15/01/19

Heilman J, 1b. https://en.wikipedia.org/wiki/Bowel_obstruction. Creative commons licence held at: https://creativecommons.org/licenses/by-sa/3.0) from Wikimedia Commons, last accessed 15/01/19

Heilman J, 1c. https://en.wikipedia.org/wiki/Inguinal_hernia#/media/File:Inquinalhernia.png Creative commons licence held at: https://creativecommons.org/licenses/by-sa/3.0), via Wikimedia Commons, last accessed 15/01/19

Heilman J, 1d. https://en.wikipedia.org/wiki/Gastrointestinal_perforation#/media/File:Free_air2010.JPG. Creative commons license held at: https://creativecommons.org/licenses/by-sa/3.0, via Wikimedia Commons, last accessed 15/01/19

Heilman J, 1e https://commons.m.wikimedia.org/wiki/File:Pancreaticpseudocyst.png#mw-jump-to-license. Creative commons license held at: https://creativecommons.org/licenses/by-sa/3.0, via Wikimedia Commons, last accessed 15/01/19

Management of acute pancreatitis. Vege SS, Whitcomb DC, Grover S. UpToDate. Last accessed 25/09/2018

Mcort NG. https://en.wikipedia.org/wiki/Anal_fistula#/media/File:Fistula_diag_01.svg. Creative commons license available at: https://creativecommons.org/licenses/by-sa/4.0, via Wikimedia Commons, last accessed 15/01/19

NIHR (National Institutes of Health) [Public domain], https://en.wikipedia.org/wiki/Inguinal_hernia#/media/File:Inguinalhernia.gif via Wikimedia Commons, last accessed 15/01/19.

Pathway for the Management of Acute Gallstone Disease. Association of Upper Gastrointestinal Surgeons of Great Britain and Ireland. Available from: http://www.augis.org/augis-guidelines/ - last accessed 15/01/19

Prognostic factors in acute pancreatitis. Blamey SL, Imrie CW, O'Neill J, Gilmour W, Carter D. Gut. 1984 25, 1340-1346

RIFT Study Group. Re-audit of the 2012 national appendicectomy audit in adults. Int J Surg. 2018;55(S1): S115.

Surgical management of the acutely obstructed colon. A review of 127 cases. Buechter KJ, Boustany C, Caillouette R, Cohn I Jr. Am J Surg. 1988 Sep;156(3 Pt 1):163-8.

Systematic review of evidence and consensus on diverticulitis: an analysis of national and international guidelines. Vennix S, Morton DG, Hahnloser D, Lange JF, Bemelman WA, Research Committee of the European Society of Coloproctology. Colorectal Dis. 2014 Nov;16(11): 866-78.

The Alvarado score for predicting acute appendicitis: a systematic review. Ohle R, O'Reilly F, O'Brien KK, Fahey T, Dimitrov B. BMC Medicine. 2011; 9(139)

The epidemiology of appendicitis and appendectomy in the United States. Addiss DG, Shaffer N, Fowler BS, Tauxe RV. Am J Epidemiol. 1990;132(5):910.

Timing and impact of infections in acute pancreatitis. Besselink MG, van Santvoort HC, Boermeester MA, Nieuwenhuijs V et al. Br J Surg. 2009 Mar;96(3):267-73. doi: 10.1002/bjs.6447.

Vaughn VM, Shuster D, Rogers MA, Mann J, Conte ML, Saint S, Chopra V. Ann Intern Med. 2017 Jun 20;166(12):883-892. doi: 10.7326/M16-2533. Epub 2017 May 16.

White Cell Count and C-Reactive Protein Measurement in Patients with Possible Appendicitis. Sengupta A, Bax G, Paterson-Brown S. Ann R Coll Surg Engl. 2009 Mar; 91(2): 113–115

Xopusmagnumx, https://commons.wikimedia.org/wiki/File:Adjustable_Gastric_Band.png. Creative commons licence held at: https://creativecommons.org/licenses/by-sa/3.0, Wikimedia Commons, last accessed 15/01/19

Wikipedia, https://commons.wikimedia.org/wiki/File:Sigmoidvolvulus.jpg. Creatice commons licence available at: https://creativecommons.org/publicdomain/zero/1.0/deed.en, via Wikimeida Commons, last accessed 20/10/2019

CHAPTER 4

ORAL AND MAXILLOFACIAL SURGERY

ZACHARY COLE-HEALY, TOBY VISHOLM & INDRAN BALASUNDARAM

Abstract
Section 1: Introduction
Scope of this chapter
Section 2: Basics
Communication
OMFS examination
Examination skills
Special test
Section 3: Trauma
General work-up
Trauma imaging
Dental trauma
Facial
Penetrating neck injuries
Fractures
Retroorbital haemorrhage
Section 4: Infections
Dento-alveolar infections
Soft Tissue infections
Section 5: Dental extraction complications
Section 6: OMFS emergencies
Airway
Massive bleeding
Carotid Blowout
Section 7: Flaps
Section 8: Important ward problems

Abstract

Oral and maxillofacial surgery (OMFS) is rarely covered in undergraduate medical training and requires both medical and dentistry degrees to enter higher training, making it very specialised. It can therefore be both daunting and challenging to junior doctors with no dentistry experience.

This chapter covers common OMFS emergency presentations and their management.

Section 1: Introduction

Scope of this chapter

Oral and Maxillofacial surgery (OMFS) is a diverse surgical specialty. It is distinct from other specialties with the requirement of dual qualification in medicine and dentistry for entry to training, in the UK (Figure 1).

Junior staff at Senior House Officer level are typically singularly qualified, either in medicine alone, or more frequently dentistry alone. Registrar level trainees will be dually qualified, however Registrars in stand-alone posts may be singularly qualified. It is therefore important to identify the background training pathways of the team you will be working with in order to work effectively and safely. Particular problems can be quite daunting to manage if they fall outside the remit of previous training; therefore one must have a low threshold for seeking senior help and support when concerned that a problem is outside of one's range of competencies.

There is also a lot of overlap between specialties: Plastic Surgery, Ear Nose and Throat Surgery and OMFS. It is important to find out on day one (or prior to starting), which specialty deals with each individual clinical presentation locally.

The purpose of this chapter is to offer an overview of the basic problems that a Senior House Officer may encounter on call, in a cross cover out of hours set up and equip them with basic knowledge to allow them to communicate clinical findings clearly to their Seniors when required.

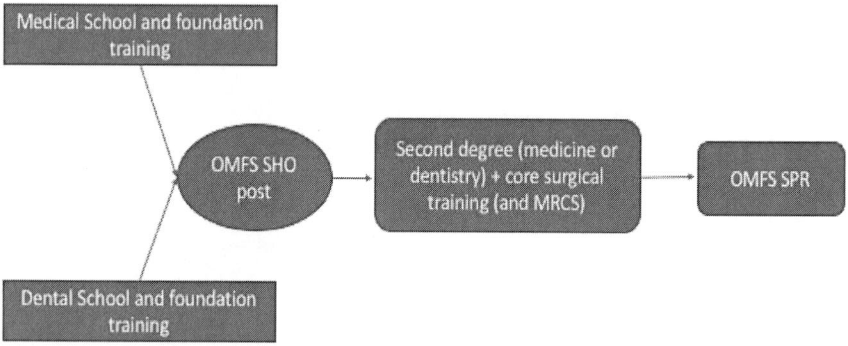

Figure 1. *Simplified training pathway for OMFS*

We will run through the basics of dentistry and OMFS examination, then common presentations to a Senior House Officer in an emergency cross cover set up.

The contents of this chapter are meant to act as a guide and draw upon our clinical experience and excellent information from other texts available on the subject (Andersson, Kahnberg, and Pogrel 2012, Braun, Marciani, and Carlson 2009, Cascarini et al. 2011, Fonseca, Barber, and Matheson 2009, Kerawala and Newlands 2014, Mitchell 2014)

Section 2: Basics

Basic dentistry

Figure 2. *Simplified tooth anatomy*
See colour centrefold for this image.

Communication

There are twenty primary (deciduous) teeth, named A-E either preceded by upper right/left or lower right/left or within a set square diagram (Figure 3).

There are 32 secondary (permanent) teeth, named 1-8 again preceded by upper right /left or lower right/left or within a set square system (Figure 3).

Dentists describe decay (caries), traumatic injuries or other dental pathology based on the surfaces that they involve.

- Mesial = towards midline
- Distal = away from midline
- Buccal = on the side of the cheek (described as labial for anterior teeth)
- Palatal = on side of palate (maxillary teeth only)
- Lingual = on side of tongue (mandibular teeth only)
- Occlusal = biting surface (described as incisal for anterior teeth)

A sound knowledge of oral and head and neck anatomy is required and there are many excellent textbooks covering this field.

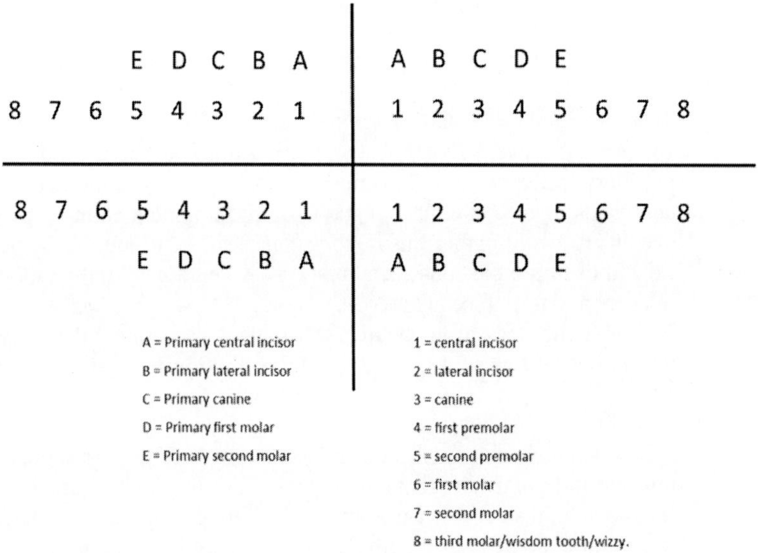

Figure 3. *Set square diagram. Imagine as if you are looking at the patient's mouth from the front*

Examination of the head and neck in the emergency department

Focus examination to the presenting complaint and history, below is a general overview:

1. Fully examine this skin of the scalp and face. Including scalp, ears, forehead, midface, nose, jaw. Note scars, lacerations, hematoma, cellulitis, asymmetry, masses and deformity.
2. Describe any lesion by site, size, shape, symmetry and surface
3. Palpate the soft tissues all over the head and face.
4. Describe any mass by temperature, consistency, fluctuance, whether fixed or mobile and other signs like associated lymphadenopathy and associated sinus.
5. Examine the facial skeleton. Note any crepitus, bruising, hematoma and lacerations. Always compare both sides of the face noting any steps in bones or deformity and asymmetry. An easy way to work is starting at the top and work down the facial skeleton.
6. Palpate the facial buttresses supraorbital rim, FZ suture, infraorbital rim, nasal bones, zygomatic arches, maxillary buttress, piriform aperture, maxillary mobility, mandible and then check the bite
7. Test the facial nerve and trigeminal nerve
8. Examine the eyes. Examine the pupils, iris and sclera. Include pupillary reflexes, eye movements, fundoscopy, fields, visual acuity (using a Snellen chart) and eye lids. If patient cannot open eye due to swelling then ensure they can see light through their eye lid and examine the consensual response when doing so. Examine the ears and nose (see chapter 2).
9. Examine the neck from behind the patient palpating bilaterally except over the carotid sinuses. Examine all lymph nodal areas.

Examination of the oral cavity:

1. Systematically examine the mucosa – including lips, buccal mucosa and gingiva, soft and hard palate, tonsils, dorsal surface of tongue, lateral sides of tongue and pull the tongue out of the mouth to examine the floor of mouth and underside of the tongue.
2. Check that there is clear saliva draining from the parotid and submandibular ducts
3. If any lesions/lacerations are identified describe their site, size, shape, surface, symmetry and palpate any lesion.
4. Palpate the cheeks, lips, tongue and with both hands, the floor of the mouth.
5. Examine the teeth systemically – start upper right last standing tooth – if required, describe any decay, fillings (restorations), or other findings such trauma (mobile teeth, fracture)

Special tests:
Percussion – if a tooth is infected and tapped firmly with a metal implement this may illicit pain. This would make it more likely that particular tooth is causing the current symptoms.

Mobility – any traumatized tooth should be examined for mobility by attempting to move it within its socket using the ends of two metal instruments. Only a very small amount of movement is physiological. Mobility can be graded 1 – 3; 0 is normal physiological movement only, 1 is small amount of lateral movement <1mm, 2 is 1-2mm lateral movement, 3 is vertical movement. Note that pre-existing mobility, secondary to periodontal (gum) disease not trauma can be present.

Flexible – nasoendoscopy – neck lumps, and orofacial infections can be from sources not visible via oral examination. Flexible nasoendoscopy can be used to identify mucosal lesions in the upper airway, or signs of epi/supra glottitis or para/retropharyngeal abscesses dependent on presentation.

Section 3: Trauma

General work up

Traumatic injuries form a large part of the emergency OMFS workload.

Assessment and treatment should be using the Advanced Trauma Life Support (ATLS) protocol. OMFS should be involved but oral-facial injuries will form part of the secondary survey. Distinct exceptions to this include any oro/facial injury which may compromise the airway, including impacted midface fractures, bilateral parasymphisis mandibular fractures, heavy oral bleeding and foreign bodies.

All patients with facial trauma must be examined by the A&E team thoroughly to clear the patient of significant head injury, cervical spine, or other injuries, prior to OMFS review. This is particularly important for OMFS as the Junior on call may be only qualified in dentistry.

Dependent on local OMFS set up, injuries can be managed in different ways. For example, most lacerations can wait until the next working day to be closed. Therefore, many units have a "hot clinic" set up and patients' wounds are cleaned overnight and they are brought back for definitive treatment during working hours. However, other departments may not have this service available and so most lacerations would be treated definitively at the time of presentation where appropriate and possible. It is therefore important to identify referral/management pathways in your local unit.

Managing OMFS presentations to the emergency department requires some specialist, sometimes hard to find, equipment including:

- Dental syringes and cartridges
- Various suture materials and sizes
- Dental splinting equipment
    - Orthodontic wire
    - Acid etch, bonding agent, dental composite, light cure
- Dental filling materials

It is therefore important to identify what is available in your department and its location, at the start of your rotation. If it is not available then, clearly, some treatments outlined below will not be possible and the patient should be redirected to where they would be available, whether that is locally at follow up, or emergency dental services.

Trauma imaging

In polytrauma and isolated significant facial trauma, ensure that the facial bones and mandible are included in the CT trauma series to prevent delays to treatment. Note that facial views and Dental Panoramic Tomography (DPT) /Ortho Pantomo Gram (OPG) imaging are not possible until the patient is able to stand, and the C-spine is cleared.

When a patient has a suspected mandibular fracture, a DPT/OPG and PA mandible should be performed. However, note that normal plain imaging does not rule out fracture particularly in the symphysis region, which is poorly imaged using the DPT and the condyles, which may be difficult to image with basic plain X-ray views.

For facial bone fractures first line plain imaging is the Occipitomental (OM) and OM30 views, which are usually described as "facial views".

Dental radiography is typically better for dental injuries, but this is unlikely to be available in the emergency department. Therefore, the DPT may be useful in ED but remember it is a higher dose of radiation for a potentially inferior image. Thus, if a minor injury then it is likely to be reasonable to wait for dental review, unless mandibular or alveolar bone fractures are suspected.

Dental trauma

Intra-oral injuries:
Tongue Lacerations: These can generally be managed conservatively. However, forked tongue, tip of tongue and lateral injuries may require repair. Discuss with a Senior if you are unsure. If repair is required, typically soft tissue infiltration with 2% lidocaine, 1/80000 adrenaline, followed by closure of the muscle layer with 3.0 non resorbable sutures e.g. vicryl, and mucosal layer with 4.0 vicryl rapide.

Pharyngeal lacerations:
These are common in children who may fall with something in their mouth – normally managed conservatively with prophylactic antibiotics but discuss with Senior as may require a CT angiogram +/- exploration. Can lead to vascular or neuronal injury if deep and delayed mediastinitis. Ensure no foreign body inhalation.

Gingival lacerations:
These are normally managed conservatively if wound edges are reasonably aligned. Beware that gingival lacerations may suggest an underlying fracture, and this should be closely examined. If closure is required typically 4.0 Vicryl Rapide single layer closure will be sufficient.

Dento-alveolar injuries:
Multiple patterns exist. Good up-to-date guidelines on management are published by the dental trauma guide online (Flores, Andreasen, and Bakland 2001).

Fractures:
May involve enamel, dentine, pulp and extend via the crown, root or both. Predominantly management should be provided by a dentist.

Ensure no foreign body inhalation or impaction in soft tissues has occurred and this may require X-ray evaluation. If pulp is not involved, then the tooth will have a good prognosis and should be seen by a dentist at the next available appointment. If the pulp is exposed, providing equipment and suitably trained staff are available it may be beneficial to treat fractured teeth with exposed pulp in the emergency department. If so, the exposed pulp is washed with sterile saline and calcium hydroxide placed over the pulp, with temporary filling material on top.

Avulsed tooth:
This is where the tooth is knocked completely out of its socket. Prognosis is dependent on time out of socket and how the tooth has been kept. Advise patient to keep the tooth in milk whilst making way to ED. Only replace adult teeth. Always ensure that the tooth is the right way around in the right socket. Ideally replantation should be performed by dentally qualified staff, however, medically qualified staff with suitable supervision are able to perform this common treatment if trained/experienced.

Management of avulsed tooth (Flores, Andreasen, and Bakland 2001):

1. Local anesthetic is given by buccal infiltration. This is where local anesthetic, typically 2% lidocaine, 1/80000 adrenaline is injected into the buccal sulcus adjacent to the tooth/tissue that needs to be anaesthetised. NB: the buccal sulcus is the space between the cheek and the alveolar bone/gingiva; the local anesthetic will diffuse through the alveolar bone to anesthetise the soft tissues, socket and teeth. Note this technique is not suitable for teeth in the posterior mandible; however, these are rarely avulsed.
2. Irrigate the socket.
3. Only ever hold the tooth by the crown.
4. Rinse the root with sterile saline.
5. Replant the tooth.
6. Get the patient to bite on gauze to hold in place.
7. Clean, rinse, acid etch, rinse, then bond the two adjacent teeth and the replanted tooth to prepare for composite bonding.
8. Splint the tooth using composite with a pre-bent orthodontic wire to one adjacent tooth either side.
9. Discharge with prophylactic antibiotics as per local guidelines. Advise urgent dental follow up; the splint should usually be removed by 2 weeks post injury.

Alveolar bone fracture:
If multiple teeth are mobile together, but the mandible/maxilla is stable, it is likely that a portion of the alveolar bone has fractured. Gingival lacerations may also be present. This may require reduction and splinting under local or general anaesthetic. Discuss with Senior if you are unsure.

Facial and neck Trauma

Soft tissue injuries

- Treatment is dependent on mechanism, wound type and anatomical location.
- Initially ATLS, ABCDE assessment and secondary survey. Rule out underlying head injury, cervical spine injury and fractures/other injuries.
- If concerned about any foreign bodies or that weapons have been used, consider radiographs of the soft tissues.
- Record all injuries and examination findings clearly in the notes in words and diagrammatically, as these may be required for future legal proceedings. Record length of wound, contamination and wound edge.
- Follow national tetanus guidelines (DOH, 2018). Generally, give Tetanus IgG + vaccine if highly contaminated wound and status unknown, or known to have no previous vaccinations and give tetanus booster injection if the patient has not had one within 10 years and relatively clean wound.

General Principles of soft tissue wound closure:

1. **Anaesthetise**: Use a mixture of local and regional anaesthetic. Local anaesthetic with adrenaline can be useful to achieve haemostasis with in the wound. Care should be taken if there is a flap of tissue with a narrow base where vasoconstriction may lead to necrosis at the tip of the flap.
2. **Assess:** Once the wound is fully anaesthetised the extent of the wound can be fully assessed as well as the degree contamination.
3. **Irrigate**: The wound should be thoroughly irrigated with normal saline, disinfected with an iodine or chlorhexidine solution followed by further irrigation with saline.
4. **Debride**: non vital tissue or badly crushed wound edges should be removed to prevent wound breakdown during healing.
5. **Haemostasis**: generally, most bleeding will have stopped prior to OMFS review. However, if this is not the case light pressure and infiltration with local with adrenaline will control generalised wound ooze. Larger vessels will require being tied off or the use of bipolar diathermy.
6. **Deep closure**: the wound should be closed in layers to prevent a hollowing deformity when the wound has healed. A 4-0 dissolvable suture should be used and one should bury the knot. **Superficial**

closure: skin should be closed with interrupted non dissolvable monofilament 5-0 sutures. The needle should pierce the skin at a 90 degree angle as this allows the curvature of the needle to ever the wound edges.

Specific laceration types

Lacerations associated with fractures

Unlike orthopedics, lacerations associated with facial fractures should be cleaned and closed as soon as possible even if the fractures are planned to be fixated electively at a later date.

Abrasions

Clean thoroughly, cover with ointment such as chloramphenicol or Vaseline and dress.

Bite injuries

Dog, cat and human bites are prone to infection. Assess tetanus risk and manage appropriately (DOH 2018). For human bites: risk assessment and consideration of HIV PEP and Hep B inoculation following local exposure guidelines. Ensure no tooth/foreign body; clean thoroughly and consider delayed closure if tissue loss, or if heavily contaminated. If deemed appropriate, primary closure and prompt emergency clinic review with prophylactic antibiotics TTO (as per local guidelines). Bite wounds and subsequent infection can cause morbidity. Therefore, if in doubt have a low threshold to discuss with Senior.

Important anatomical considerations for facial laceration management

Prior to any closure one must fully examine the facial nerve function and if there is any deficit this should be discussed with a Senior, as it is likely to need exploration and closure in theatre. A useful landmark is a straight vertical line running down from the lateral border of the eye. Any nerve injury lateral to this should be explored in theatre with a microscope and an attempt to coapt the nerve should be pursued. Medial to this landmark, the nerve is deemed too small to identify.

There is much overlap between specialties (OMFS, ENT, Plastics, Ophthalmology) when dealing with facial lacerations. Local arrangements usually exist to dictate to which team these should be referred and treated, so find these out. If unsure, regarding best management, discuss with your Senior and consider discussion with other specialties as required.

Some important anatomical areas to note:

- Eye-lid: only repair if confident and experienced. Rule out associated globe injury. A general rule is if it is superficial and involves skin only, OMFS will close. If through and through, muscle or tarsal plate involvement this will warrant referral to ophthalmology for closure, as inappropriate management can lead to significant morbidity.
- Ears: consider referral, or at least discussion, with ENT. Remember the cartilage is avascular and requires adjacent skin for blood supply or it will become necrotic/inflamed (cauliflower ear); therefore, always drain pinna haematomas, ensuring that all cartilage is covered after closure and dress with pressure to prevent haematoma accumulation. Generally, management includes deep cartilage approximation and skin closure with non-resorbable sutures e.g. 5.0 prolene.
- Nose: consider referral or discussion with ENT. If full thickness, close the inner mucosal layer first, ensuring cartilage is covered. If tissue loss, or deep injury consult Senior and probably ENT will require delayed reconstruction.
- Cheek: Prior to closure, examine the parotid duct intraorally (on the buccal surface of the cheek generally adjacent to the second molar.) If any blood can be milked into the duct, this suggests injury and should be discussed with a Senior as these generally will be closed in theatre. Examine the facial nerve fully prior to local anaesthetic, as described above.
- Lips: if through and through – align vermillion border with one non resorbable suture e.g 5.0 prolene. Close muscle layer with resorbable sutures e.g vicryl 3.0; close mucosal layer with resorbable sutures (E.g 4.0 or 5.0 vicryl rapide), then close the skin with non-resorbable (E.g 5.0 or 6.0 prolene).

Fractures

Information presented below is an overview. For further information please review Oxford Handbook of Oral and Maxillofacial surgery (Cascarini et al. 2011). For on-the-go advice and in depth information the textbook of Oral and Maxillofacial surgery (Braun, Marciani, and Carlson 2009, Fonseca, Barber, and Matheson 2009) is recommended.

Mandibular fractures:
These are one of the most common referrals and operations performed by the OMFS team.

Fully assess the patient as there may be other injuries. Be sure to identify head and cervical spine injury. Beware of significant intra-oral swelling where hematoma in the sublingual space bilaterally can present with airway compromise. Also, beware of bilateral symphysis/para-symphysis fractures where the tongue loses anterior attachment and can occlude the airway.

- Symptoms: Pain, swelling, teeth not meeting normally, numbness of the lower lip/chin (indicates damage to the inferior alveolar nerve which runs in canal in the mandible). Any numbness should be clearly documented as this is also a possible complication due to fracture reduction and fixation.
- Signs: Malocclusion; step deformity at the site of fracture; overlying lacerations; mobile teeth/segment; numbness; trismus and haematoma. (Andersson, Kahnberg, and Pogrel 2012)
- Diagnosis: DPT and PA mandible or CT facial bones.
- Management:
    - Most fractures will require admission and open reduction with internal fixation the next day. Occasionally non-displaced, non-mobile favourable fractures, including unilateral condylar fractures can be managed conservatively, but only allow this management if advised by a Senior.
    - Admission. NBM. Antibiotics (as per local guidelines), if any dental involvement or associated laceration intra-orally. Place on emergency list or theatre list available the next day. Admission bloods. Analgesia. IV Fluids.

Zygomatic fractures:
These classically present as a tripod fracture with fracture at the zygomatic arch, zygomatic-frontal suture and orbital rim. However, multiple fracture patterns exist. The key point is to consider the presence of retrobulbar haemorrhage (see below) and treat urgently if present.

- Symptoms/signs: deformity of the cheek, tender zygomatic-frontal suture, bony step, eye injuries particularly subconjunctival haemorrhage with no posterior limit, numbness to cheek and lip, epistaxis and trismus (Braun, Marciani, and Carlson 2009). If there is mobility of the maxilla then suspect a Le-Fort midface fracture.
- Examination of the eye is paramount

- Diagnosis: OM and OM30 if complicated. CT facial bones may be required.
- Management: Any associated ocular injury should be reviewed by ophthalmology, if no retrobulbar haemorrhage then OPD review in 1 week is normally acceptable with definitive surgical treatment within 14 days. Advise patients not to blow their nose. Consider prophylactic antibiotics: follow local advice regarding this.

Orbital floor fractures:
Any part of the orbital rim which is made up of multiple bones may fracture. However, the orbital floor being thinnest, is more frequently fractured.

- Beware of retrobulbar haemorrhage (see below) which though more common in zygomatic fractures can occur with orbital floor fractures.
- Especially in children (but also in adults), it is important to assess for a trap door fracture where blood supply to the inferior rectus muscle is compromised by the fracture segment, leading to subsequent necrosis. This can lead to significant morbidity and must not be missed. This is presented with severe pain and ophthalmoplegia to upward gaze. If concerned, CT and discuss with Senior urgently.
- Symptoms/Signs: Diplopia, subconjunctival haemorrhage, tenderness, numbness, bruising, exophthalmos. Enopthalmos (globe moves posteriorly) and hypoglobus (globe moves inferiorly), as the swelling subsides, can present in a delayed fashion (Braun, Marciani, and Carlson 2009).
- Diagnosis: OM / OM 30. If indicated prior to surgical repair, CT facial bones/orbit is likely to be required.
- Management:
    - Discuss with ophthalmology or refer as per local pathways. The urgency of ophthalmology review will be guided by signs and symptoms. They will arrange for orthoptic assessment if diplopia is present, prior to surgical repair.
    - Children have a higher incidence of trap door fractures and usually should be discussed with a Senior prior to discharge.
    - Arrange follow up in clinic within 1 week.
    - Patient should not blow their nose.
    - Consider antibiotic prophylaxis as per local guidelines.

Retrobulbar haemorrhage:
This can be considered as a compartment syndrome of the eye. Bleeding increases pressure which leads to a loss of blood supply to the optic nerve and blindness. **Aim is for prompt diagnosis and management to prevent visual loss.**

It can occur following trauma in fractures involving the orbit or surgical procedures to the orbit. It classically presents with loss of visual acuity with one or more of the following: pain, proptosis, ophthalmoplegia, hard globe, loss of direct pupillary reflex. All features may not be present; therefore, a high index of suspicion must be maintained when reviewing patients with orbital trauma, particularly if patient is intubated (Cascarini et al. 2011).

Management involves prompt surgical treatment with adjunctive medical treatment which allows time for definitive treatment.

Surgical management consists of lateral canthotomy and cantholysis which should only be performed by suitably trained and experienced staff (they may be from A&E, OMFS or Ophthalmology specialties). It can be performed under LA or GA. It is a temporizing treatment that increases orbital volume. Definitive treatment will then need to be planned. Medical management includes topical timolol, IV steroids, IV Mannitol, IV Acetazolamide (Cascarini et al. 2011).

If a patient is already intubated then diagnosis based on visual acuity is not possible so urgent Senior advice should be sought, if there is any clinical suspicion. CT orbit may be required.

Maxillary fractures:
Fracture patterns are historically described using the Le-Fort categorization. Beware of airway compromise from a posteriorly impacted midface fracture. Also, be wary of CSF leak from associated base of skull fracture (Andersson, Kahnberg, and Pogrel 2012).

- Signs/Symptoms: Midface mobility based on level of fracture. Palatal laceration if associated palatal fracture. Lengthening of the face. Racoon eyes.
- Diagnosis: OM/OM30. If Le-Fort fracture suspected, then CT facial bones will be required. Le-Fort fracture hallmark is pterygomaxillary separation.

  - Le-fort 1 – Known as a floating palate - Horizontal fracture at the level of the nasal floor leading to mobile palate and alveolar bone.
  - Le-fort 2 – Known as pyramidal fracture – level of fracture at the inferior orbital rim and down the medial wall of the maxillary sinus.
  - Le-fort 3 – Known as cranio-facial dissociation – level of fracture at the zygomatic arch and naso-frontal suture.
- Management:
  - Admission.
  - ATLS - ABCDE
  - Dis-impaction and nasal packing as required.
  - NBM. Pre-op work up.
  - ORIF is usually delayed if the patient is comfortable and there is no acute airway or bleeding issue.

Nasal fracture:

Nasal fractures are common and generally only require management if there are functional or aesthetic complications. However, in the emergency setting one must rule out head injury and deal with immediate complications. These may be followed up by OMFS or ENT dependent on local referral pathways.

- Signs and symptoms: bruising, epistaxis, deformity of bridge or nasal septum, swelling. Note that nasal fracture may be associated with septal hematoma.
- Diagnosis: clinical, however OM/OM30, CT head and or facial bones, may be required to rule out other injuries.
- Management: If no major aesthetic or functional concern, GP review within 7 days may be suitable. If likely to require MUA, or unsure, then arrange emergency clinic appointment in 1 week. Note, MUA, if required, must be performed within 14 days.

- Epistaxis: This can be severe and life threatening. Immediate first aid with pressure bilaterally on the soft part of the anterior nose will usually stop the bleeding. However, anterior/posterior nasal packing may be required (See chapter 2).

Septal hematoma:

This involves bilateral swelling of the anterior nasal septum, as the septum derives its blood supply from the mucosa. This can lead to cartilaginous necrosis and collapse of the nose leading to poor aesthetics and difficult surgical repair. If identified, discuss with Senior as it will require emergency drainage, usually by ENT.

Nasoethmoidal fracture:
Nasal fractures which extend to the cranium and orbital walls (Mitchell 2014).

- Signs and symptoms: upturned nose, flattened nasal bridge, traumatic telecanthus, CSF rhinorrhea, panda eyes, nasal blockage and blocked nasolacrimal ducts.
- Management: treat associated lacerations and injuries. Arrange for CT imaging. Discuss with Senior. ORIF is normally done electively.

Frontal sinus fracture:
It is important not to miss this and if there is any suspicion, perform a CT head.

- Anterior wall: depression will likely cause aesthetic compromise but no other long or short-term complications. Give antibiotics and arrange urgent OPD follow up.
- Posterior wall: complicated management and high risk of neurological complications. Admit. IV antibiotics. Neurological examination. Discuss with Senior.

TMJ Dislocation:
This may be caused by any incident that leads to hyper-extension of the TMJ. It is more common in patients with hyper-mobility syndrome.

Diagnosis is clinical, with imaging being supportive when evaluating for differential diagnosis of displaced fracture.

- TMJ reduction:
    - Avoid sedation
    - Pressure bilaterally on the lower molars pushing inferiorly; simultaneously close the anterior mandible. Alternatively, the patient can bite with the molars on a 10ml syringe, with simultaneous closing of the anterior mandible.

- o Avoid excessive force.
- o Multiple failed attempts suggest that reduction under general anaesthetic may be required.

Section 4: Infections

Dento-alveolar infections

Toothache is a common presentation to ED, particularly at night and weekend when emergency dental services are not available. It is inappropriate for OMFS to review all patients presenting with toothache. They should be assessed and discharged with analgesia and information on how to access local dental services.

However, dento-alveolar infections that have spread from the tooth into the surrounding tissues represent an emergency with multiple possible complications. Treatment is drainage of abscess, removal of source of infection (tooth) and antibiotics to stabilise condition.

Consider differential diagnosis, particularly for infections of ENT origin, including tonsillitis, peritonsillar abscess, para/retropharyngeal abscess, supra and epiglottitis (See chapter 2). Infection of the salivary glands and infected sebaceous cysts will also present similarly. They may be managed by ENT or OMFS dependent on local referral pathways.

Important markers from history and examination that are of concern include: (Cascarini et al. 2011)

- Airway compromise – cellulitis of the soft tissues supporting the upper airway can occlude this space rapidly leading to the loss of the airway.
- Raised floor of mouth and difficulty with tongue protrusion may suggest swelling or abscess of the sublingual space.
- Change in voice, difficulty swallowing, or painful swallowing and drooling are very concerning signs for impending airway compromise.
- Systemic inflammatory response syndrome – indicates sepsis as source of infection is present and should therefore be treated with the sepsis care bundle in addition to source control.
- Ludwigs angina – this is pan-cellulitis of the sublingual and submandibular spaces bilaterally. The neck usually appears tense

and swollen and the floor of the mouth is raised or firm. There may be swallowing difficulty and a soft stridor. This is a true surgical emergency. ABCDE management, urgent anaesthetic and Senior review enabling immediate treatment, is required.

- Midface infection – the cerebral veins do not have valves so any cellulitis involving the nasal or orbital region can therefore spread via this venous route and potentially cause cavernous sinus thrombosis.
- Peri-orbital cellulitis – typically caused by sinusitis and managed by the ENT team. However, infection of maxillary canine teeth can lead to this. Treatment is by IV antibiotics, I&D of abscess and extraction of causative teeth.
- Untreated infections may spread via the fascial spaces to the mediastinum causing mediastinitis.

Management:

- Definitive airway if required/anaesthetics review
- High flow oxygen if airway compromise
- IV Access.
- Bloods (FBC UE CRP INR BM Cultures G&S)
- IV antibiotics +/- IV Steroids as per local guidelines
- IV fluids
- NBM
- DPT/ OPG
- CT (or ultrasound) may be required - discuss with Senior.

Section 5: Dental Extraction Complications

Bleeding:

- Bleeding post extraction is an important and common problem.
- Any socket can bleed even with simple extractions.
- The responsible socket should be quickly identified by oral examination; however, the precise bleeding point may be difficult to identify and may be deep to the visible tissue.
- The patient should be asked to bite down on a wet gauze pack placed over the socket for 10 minutes. This may be soaked in adrenaline or tranexamic acid to aid haemostasis. Concurrently buccal infiltration and infiltration of the soft tissues with lidocaine 2% with 1/80000 adrenaline should be performed.
- The above methods should reduce or cease bleeding.

- Definitive management may include packing the socket with an oxidised cellulose haemostat and performing a mattress suture, or two simple interrupted sutures, across the socket to provide tension.
- If there is ongoing bleeding despite the above treatment, consider discussion with Senior. Subsequent management may include diathermy, bone wax and other techniques.
- Consider checking patients FBC and clotting. Consider discharging with antibiotics if delayed (>24 hours) haemorrhage. Always give the patient a sterile pack of gauze to take home in case of further bleeding and contact details/plan of what to do if it recurs.

Dry socket:
This is pain which becomes severe 3-5 days following extraction. Normally bone is visible in the socket which is devoid of blood clot. Management is simple analgesia along with irrigation of the socket with saline and packing with an obtundent dressing, e.g. alvogyl, which can normally be provided during dental follow up.

Hematoma:
This is common. Assess for airway compromise but most can be managed conservatively. Seek Senior help if unsure.

Infection:
This is uncommon. Consider radiograph to rule out retained root. Drain collections if present. Clean/irrigate the socket. Prescribe antibiotics.

Oro-antral communication:
This is a hole between the upper socket and the maxillary sinus. Arrange follow up in the clinic. Definitive closure can be done under local anaesthetic. Give the patient antibiotics and advise no nose blowing in the meantime. Consider CT imaging to confirm the diagnosis.

Numbness:
Common following extraction of lower molars – normally resolves but can take many months. Arrange follow up.

Section 6: Emergencies

Airway problems

Manage as per ABCDE or ATLS protocol dependent on the mechanism. Seek urgent Senior and anaesthetics support.

Trauma:
In facial trauma, often severe bleeding from the orofacial region will compromise the airway. This is likely to occur before C Spine clearance. Consider log roll to allow patient to spit blood out until a definitive airway can be achieved. Midface fractures and mandible fractures can be depressed and compromise the airway. Airway adjuncts and physical manipulation of the depressed fracture segments may be required. Prior to intubation, identification of staff to perform surgical cricothyroidotomy, if required, is paramount. In laryngeal trauma, surgical tracheostomy may be preferred to cricothyroidotomy. Discuss with ENT.

Post-operative expanding neck:
In post-operative patients, hematoma can compromise the airway. Sit the patient forward, administer oxygen, consider removal of the sutures and drainage of the clot. Arrange for urgent Senior review and anesthetics support.

Infections:
In patients with orofacial infection and signs of impending or actual airway compromise, arrange for urgent Senior and anaesthetics review; ensure theatre is aware of the case. Urgent definitive airway via intubation (typically nasal or surgical) is the primary treatment, followed by drainage of abscess, antibiotics and steroids.

Tracheostomy patient: See chapter 2

Massive bleeding

Bleeding from the neck:
Penetrating neck injuries associated with heavy bleeding should be managed with an ATLS resuscitation, together with prompt Senior and anaesthetics review. Whilst traditionally all penetrating neck injuries deep of platysma must be surgically explored, in current practice, CT angiography is now frequently used if patient is asymptomatic and stable.

For descriptive purposes injuries are typically described based on anatomical level (Brennan and Holt 2012).

- Level 1 – Clavicle to cricoid
- Level 2 – Cricoid to the mandible
- Level 3 – From mandible to base of the skull

If CT angiography is performed and is normal, be aware this does not have 100% sensitivity and that trachea-oesophageal injuries may not be identified. Seek urgent Senior review.

Carotid blowout:
If predicted, for example in palliative cancer patient, follow pre-agreed management plan using palliative medications available.

If not expected, manage as per ABCDE. Be aware of patients DNAR status. Apply pressure to bleeding point. Put out a crash call, arrange urgent Senior review as appropriate, resuscitate but do not delay getting the patient to theatre.

Bleeding from the face/nose:
Common causes include facial trauma, with bleeding secondary to lacerations, or fractures and epistaxis which may or may not be traumatic.

Be aware it is easy to underestimate blood loss as some may be swallowed/concealed and proper resuscitation must be instigated for all patients with significant bleeding.

If possible, sit the patient up and use high volume suction; try to identify the bleeding point.

Midface fracture bleeding:
Posterior and anterior nasal packing, then impact the mid face by getting the patient to bite on gauze. This may be difficult if there is a concurrent mandibular fracture.

Mandibular fracture bleeding:
Beware of concealed bleeding in the floor of the mouth which may present with airway compromise. Seek urgent Senior review.

Bleeding from laceration:
Lacerations may rupture the superficial arteries of the face including the superficial temporal artery and facial arteries. Stem bleeding with pressure. **Examine for facial nerve injury and other associated injuries prior to local anaesthetic.** Anaesthetise the area. If possible to identify the bleeding point, then clip and tie, or consider large tacking sutures to tamponade the bleeding temporarily. Otherwise wait for Senior help.

Non-traumatic epistaxis: See chapter 2

Section 7: Flaps

Flaps will be covered in more depth in chapter 6. However, it is important to remember that both free and pedicle flaps can fail. In free flaps, most commonly, failure is due to venous compromise at the anastomosis and less commonly arterial. Manage with an ABCDE approach as a deteriorating patient is unlikely to have a healthy flap. Differential diagnosis of anastomotic flap failure includes haematoma and shock.

Flap failure is an emergency. Delayed identification can lead to significant morbidity. Communicate your assessment to a Senior urgently and if advised, prepare for theatre.

Assessment of flap: ABCDE assessment, review the flap monitoring chart and discuss with nursing staff re their concerns. Examine the flap for colour, warmth, CRT, doppler anastomosis (handheld - usually marked at the time of surgery, or internal probe placed during surgery), evaluate for haematoma, review drain output, ensure no compression of neck by dressing/ties, put the head in a neutral position (Cascarini, 2018).

Herald bleed from flap
Bleeding from a flap may lead to haematoma and subsequent vascular compromise at the anastomosis/pedicle. If identified, the flap should be closely monitored and Senior review sought as the patient may require re-exploration urgently.

Section 8: Important ward problems

Drain not working

Generally, drains are removed when output is less than 20ml/24 hours. Typically drains will drain for the first 24 hours and then drainage will slow, and they will be removed. However, if nothing is being drained, particularly during the first 24 hours, the drain may not be working properly. Differential includes blockage, leakage (of vacuum seal) or dislodgement. Examine the neck, ensure the drain tie is intact and ask the nursing staff to confirm that the vacuum is effective. Discuss with Senior, as the drain may need to be removed slightly or, in the context of significant swelling, replaced.

References

Andersson, Lars, Karl-Erik Kahnberg, and M Anthony Pogrel. 2012. *Oral and maxillofacial surgery*: John Wiley & Sons.

Braun, Thomas, Robert Marciani, and Eric Carlson. 2009. *Oral and Maxillofacial Surgery - Trauma, Surgical Pathology, Temporomadibular Disorders.* Edited by Robert Marciani. Second ed. 2 vols. Vol. 2. Missouri Saunders.

Brennan, Joseph , and Richard Holt. 2012. *Resident Manual of Trauma to the Face, Head and Neck* Edited by Richard Holt: American Academy of Otolarngology - Head and Neck Surgery Foundation.

Cascarini, Luke, Clare Schilling, Ben Gurney, and Peter Brennan. 2011. *Oxford Handbook of Oral and Maxillofacial Surgery*. Oxford: Oxford University Press.

DOH. 2018 Immunisation Green Book: Chapter 30: Tetanus. edited by Department-of-Health. London: Department-of-Health

Flores, MT, JO Andreasen, and LK Bakland. 2001. "Guidelines for the evaluation and Management of traumatic dental injuriesEditors Note." *Dental traumatology* 17 (5):193-196.

Fonseca, Raymond, Dexter Barber, and John Matheson. 2009. *Oral and Maxillofacial Surgery - Anaesthesia and pain control, Dentoalveolar Surgery, Practice Management, Implant Surgery.* Edited by Raymond Fonseca. 2 ed. 3 vols. Vol. One, *Oral and Maxillofacial Surgery* Missouri Saunders.

Kerawala, Cyrus, and Carrie Newlands. 2014. *Oral and maxillofacial surgery*: OUP Oxford.

Mitchell, David A. 2014. *An introduction to oral and maxillofacial surgery*: Oxford University Press.

CHAPTER 5

PAEDIATRIC SURGERY

SIMON MCCLUNEY & IAIN YARDLEY

Abstract
Section 1 – Herniae
Inguinal Herniae
Umbilical Herniae
Section 2 – Scrotal Pathology
Hydrocele
Testicular torsion
Torted Appendix Testis
Section 3 – Pyloric stenosis
Section 4 – Appendicitis
Section 5 – Intussusception
Section 6 – Neonates
Obstruction
Malrotation
Hirschsprung disease
Necrotising enterocolitis
Tracheo-oesophageal fistula
Section 7 – Practical skills
Feeding tubes
Intravenous access
Local Aesthetic
Blood sampling
Section 8 – Prescribing
Neonatal fluids
Conclusion

Abstract

Paediatric surgery offers a unique set of pathologies and challenges for the junior doctor cross-covering on call. The key to successfully negotiating an on call covering paediatric surgery is to be able to take a history and examine a child and pass the relevant information onto your senior colleagues who will support you in decision making. It is necessary to have a broad understanding of paediatric surgical pathologies as then you will be able to identify them and begin to formulate appropriate management plans for children of all ages.

This chapter will cover key paediatric surgical pathologies, their presentation and management. It will also cover key principles for paediatric prescribing and offer tips for practical skills needed in paediatric surgery, including cannulating and blood taking.

Section 1: Herniae

Inguinal Herniae

Primary inguinal hernias occur in 1-5% of new-borns, rising to approximately 10% in those born prematurely (Grosfeld 1989, 506). Inguinal herniae in children are almost exclusively indirect hernias due to a failure of the processus vaginalis to obliterate, allowing communication between the inguinal canal and the abdominal cavity. Surgical repair consists of high ligation and excision of the processus vaginalis, without the use of a mesh. Right sided herniae are more common, as the left processus vaginalis obliterates before the right in utero. There is, however, a 5-20% chance of developing a contralateral hernia.

History and Examination

The commonest presentation is with an intermittent bulge associated with times of increased abdominal pressure, leading to crying. Patients should be examined both lying down and standing. The typical location of the bulge is above and medial to the pubic tubercle and in boys this may extend into the scrotum. Occasionally, no swelling is elicited on examination despite a good history of a hernia being given and in this case other signs can be useful. The spermatic cord on the affected side may feel thicker than the contralateral side and rubbing the cord structures against the pubic tubercle is said to feel like two layers of silk rubbing against each other in the presence of a hernia: the "silk glove sign". Where a scrotal swelling is found, the key differential is a hydrocoele. Classically, you cannot "get above" a hernia as it is continuous with the processus vaginalis, whereas you usually can with a hydrocoele (see below). Transillumination can be useful to differentiate between a hydrocoele and a hernia; it is usually present in hydrocoeles and not with hernias. However, one must demonstrate some caution as both can transilluminate in very young patients. Ultrasound scanning can be useful in equivocal cases.

In girls, the intra-abdominal contents herniate via the canal of Nuck, which is analogous to the processus vaginalis. This connects the peritoneal cavity to the labia majora, thus an inguinal hernia is an important differential diagnosis for the unilateral swollen labium.

Complications

Clinical examination is paramount, and different clinicians can sometimes appear to use terms such as incarceration with different meanings. Incarceration is the trapping of hernia contents preventing reduction, i.e. an irreducible hernia. Strangulation is loss of blood supply to the hernia contents, resulting in ischaemia and necrosis. In the paediatric population, the incidence of incarceration is approximately 15-30% and incarceration is a clinical diagnosis (Puri, Guiney, O'Donnell 1984, 44).

Management

If a simple, easily reducible, inguinal hernia is diagnosed, the child should have elective surgical repair as soon as practical to avoid complications. In infants <1kg inguinal herniae are present in 30% and can be safely monitored as long as the hernia is reducible, with planned repair once the child reaches around 2kg (Peevy, Speed, Hoff 1986, 246).

Patients with an incarcerated hernia should have attempted reduction with analgesia and/or sedation in the emergency department, and if successful proceeding to expedited surgical repair within 48 hours. If unsuccessful, they require urgent surgery. With appropriate analgesia and a skilled operator, the vast majority of hernias are reducible in the emergency department (Bowling, Hart, Cox, Srinivas 2017, 4484). Reduction is achieved by gentle constant pressure on the distal aspect of the hernia – guiding it along the direction of the inguinal canal and through the superficial and deep inguinal rings. In female patients, reduction should be more gentle, due to the risk of reproductive organs being present in the hernia sac.

Umbilical Herniae

Umbilical herniae occur due to the passage of the umbilical vessels through the umbilical ring in-utero. They should be considered a normal finding in the infant period. In white patients, they affect approximately 10-30% of new-borns, reducing to 2-10% at 1 year; whilst rates in the African population have been estimated at 23-85% (Bowling, Hart, Cox, Srinivas 2017, 4484).

Presentation

These children will typically present with a painless lump in the umbilicus, with increased protrusion when crying or straining. They can appear very large which is often a concern for parents, although the defect is usually relatively small. They very rarely cause symptoms and studies have demonstrated a rate of incarceration of approximately one in 1500 (Bowling, Hart, Cox, Srinivas 2017, 4484).

Management

The vast majority will resolve spontaneously as the umbilical ring closes by the age of five. Therefore, children with an umbilical hernia can be discharged from surgical follow up and re-referred if the hernia persists when they are 4. The parents should be safety netted to seek medical advice if the hernia is ever very painful, tender, irreducible or develops skin changes. After 4-5 years of age, elective surgery is recommended. In rare cases of incarceration, manual reduction should be attempted using similar techniques to those described for inguinal herniae. If successful, the hernia should be repaired within 48 hours of presentation. If it is truly irreducible, urgent surgery is required.

Section 2: Scrotal Pathology

Groin and testicular swellings make up a large proportion of the workload of a paediatric surgical unit, both emergent and elective. Diagnosis can be much more challenging than in the adult population, and you must maintain a high degree of suspicion when assessing these children.

Hydrocoele

A hydrocoele is a collection of peritoneal fluid between the parietal and visceral layers of the tunica vaginalis. In childhood the vast majority are communicating hydrocoeles due to a failure of closure of the processus vaginalis.

Presentation

Patients present with a scrotal mass that changes in size during the day, or on Valsalva, but are often reducible. Differentiating a hydrocoele from a hernia can be difficult for those with limited experience but it is usually possible to "get above" a hydrocoele and palpate the spermatic cord superior to the scrotal swelling and hydrocoeles will typically brightly transilluminate, when a pen torch is shone through the scrotum. However, if there is any doubt Senior support should be sought.

Management

Generally speaking infants under 2 years of age can be discharged as the majority of hydrocoeles will resolve spontaneously in time. If a child present with a hydrocoele at an external hospital, they do not need to be seen urgently and can be referred to an outpatient clinic. This requires, however, that the referring clinician is confident in the diagnosis. If there is uncertainty, they should be seen by a specialist. If a hydrocoele persists beyond the age of 2, surgical intervention is indicated with a PPV ligation, as for an inguinal hernia.

Testicular torsion

The acute scrotum is a common referral to paediatric surgery centres, and as the SHO on call, you should take all such referrals as a priority. Testicular torsion is an acute surgical emergency and, where suspected, patients should have operative management within 6 hours to try and salvage the testicle. The peak incidence of testicular torsion is in adolescence, with a small peak in the neonatal period.

History

The classical presentation is acute onset severe testicular/scrotal pain which may radiate to the abdomen or groin. The majority have associated nausea and vomiting, whilst some patients may have intermittent pain, if the testicle is repeatedly torting and detorting.

Examination

On examination, the affected side is usually obvious with scrotal swelling and erythema. The testicle may lie higher in the scrotum due to cord shortening and have a more "horizontal" lie than normal. In delayed presentations, a reactive hydrocoele may be present. The cremasteric reflex is normally absent in torsion. This is tested by gently stroking the superomedial aspect of the thigh. In a normal scenario, the ipsilateral testicle should move superiorly due to contraction of the cremaster muscle.

Investigations

The diagnosis is clinical, and no investigations are routinely required. In patients with either suspected testicular torsion, or where a torsion cannot be excluded, the next step must be an emergent scrotal exploration. Even if the history is prolonged, surgery should never be delayed, as the testicle cannot be presumed to be non-viable. The role of ultrasonography is limited and should only be performed if the test will not delay surgery. It is mostly utilised for those patients who have suffered testicular trauma, to rule out a tunica rupture, haematoma or haematocele.

Management

As the SHO, your job is to identify this referral as a high priority, assess and examine the patient and escalate early to the Registrar. If you are confident in the diagnosis, consenting the patient, contacting theatres and the on-call anaesthetic team should be done simultaneously to avoid delay. Even in cases where you are sure it is not a testicular torsion, having a low threshold for Senior involvement is advised.

Surgical preference depends on the responsible clinician. In most centres, if the testicle is normal, and the pathology was, for example, a torted appendix testis, the contralateral side does not have to be explored. However, if the testicle was torted, the contralateral side should also be fixed. This is because the bell clapper deformity (where the testis lacks normal attachment to tunica vaginalis and lies horizontally, so predisposing to torsion), is often bilateral when present. Surgical preference differs on how to fix a testis. Clear instructions should be gained from the senior surgeon before the operation begins.

Torted Appendix Testis

The appendix testis, or hydatid of Morgagni, is a vestigial remnant of the Mullerian system and is present in 90% of patients. It is located at the head of the epididymis and it can also undergo torsion. In these patients, **the testicle body should be non-tender**, with a focally tender area at the superior or inferior pole. If the appendix testis is gangrenous, it may appear as a "blue dot" through the scrotal skin although this is hard to elicit in non-

Caucasian patients. If the clinician is extremely confident in the diagnosis, these patients are managed conservatively, with surgical excision of the torted appendix only if the pain is persistent. However, if there is any doubt in the diagnosis the child should be managed as a testicular torsion and an emergent scrotal exploration performed. Again, in such patients, review by a Senior surgeon should be sought.

Section 3: Pyloric Stenosis

Infantile hypertrophic pyloric stenosis occurs typically within the first few weeks of life and is rare after 3 months. It is much more common in boys than girls and a positive family history is often present.

Presentation

Classically, the infant is a "**hungry vomiter**", with **forceful non-bilious vomiting after each feed and wanting to be re-fed immediately after**. The vomiting is typically forceful and occurs immediately after feeding, helping to distinguish it from reflux. Babies with pyloric stenosis are often dehydrated and will usually have had some weight loss. There may be a palpable pyloric tumour in the right upper quadrant, said to feel like "an olive under a blanket". Infants who present late will have the classic hypochloraemic, hypokalaemic, metabolic alkalosis.

Investigation

The palpation of an olive-like mass on clinical examination with a typical history is diagnostic, but ultrasonography is commonplace and usually utilised. On ultrasonography, the classical pathological dimensions are typically regarded as pyloric muscle thickness (single wall) greater than 3mm, and a length greater than 15mm (Rohrschneider, Mittnacht, Darge 1998, 429-34).

Management

The child should be made nil by mouth and a nasogastric tube (10 or 12 Fr) inserted and placed on free drainage with hourly aspirations. Routine blood tests, including a blood gas, should be obtained. The child should be resuscitated if dehydrated, using 0.9% saline boluses of 10ml/kg, until the heart rate and capillary refill return to normal. Electrolyte losses should then be corrected with maintenance fluid of 10% glucose, 0.9% saline and 10mmol KCl per 500ml, at a rate of 150ml/kg/day. Nasogastric losses should be replaced ml for ml with normal saline with potassium. Blood gases should be performed every 12 hours to assess biochemical status.

Definitive treatment is with a surgical pyloromyotomy, where the pyloric muscle is split leaving the underlying mucosa intact. This can only be safely undertaken when the electrolytes and acid-base balance have returned to normal. This may take several days, and the priority of initial management is careful fluid replacement and monitoring of the electrolyte abnormalities. Surgery can be performed via a variety of incisions or laparoscopically (Downey 1998, 220; Perger, Fuchs, Komidar, Mooney 2009, 2119). Feeding can be slowly introduced on the operative day in a stepwise fashion and the infant discharged when tolerating full feeds.

Section 4: Appendicitis

Appendicitis is the most common general surgical pathology in childhood. It presents most frequently in the second decade of life. **Care must be taken when assessing those of pre-school age, as they often present with non-specific symptoms**. Indeed, studies have shown perforation rates to be as high as 83% in neonates and 51% in those under 5 years old, whereas this drops to 10-20% in those over 12 (Schwartz, Gilad, Sigalet, Yu et al. 2011, 2060-2064; Horwitz, Gursoy, Jaksic, Lally 1997, 80; Nance, Adamson, Hedrick 2006, 160; Colvin, Bachur, Kharbanda 2007, 849-855; Addiss, Shaffer, Fowler, Tauxe 1990, 910)

History & Examination

The classic history of anorexia with migration of periumbilical pain to the right iliac fossa is not as common in children as in adults; whilst those under 5 years old may present in many ways including being non-specifically unwell. Clinical examination is key, and like adults, local tenderness with peritonism near McBurney's point is the most reliable sign.

Investigations

Blood tests are important adjuncts but should always be taken in context with the clinical picture. When the white cell count and the C-reactive protein are both raised, the specificity is approximately 90% (Kwan, Nager 2010, 1009-1015). The Paediatric Appendicitis Score (PAS) and the Alvarado score are two scoring systems for appendicitis that are commonly used but neither is wholly reliable.

For children without a typical presentation, imaging can be a useful diagnostic adjunct. Ultrasound is the most commonly used test and is readily accessible without the risk of radiation. The accuracy of the test, however, is dependent on the operator performing the scan, in addition to the body habitus of the patient. Computed tomography can be used, but due to the associated radiation, is a Senior led decision and should not be requested by junior staff members.

Management

There are a multitude of alternative diagnoses, the most common of which are mesenteric adenitis, gastroenteritis and urinary tract infections. If there is diagnostic uncertainty and the child is systemically well, an observational approach may be adopted with serial examinations until a diagnosis can be established. If the child is being treated for appendicitis, they should receive analgesia, intravenous fluids for resuscitation, antibiotics and operative management.

The operative approach to appendicectomy depends on the centre and can be performed by open surgery, or laparoscopically. Laparoscopic appendicectomy is associated with a reduced length of hospital stay compared to open surgery, with small differences in post-operative complications between the two, with a large meta-analysis demonstrating laparoscopic procedures are associated with a lower risk of wound infection but a higher risk of intra-abdominal abscesses (Markar, Blackburn, Cobb, Karthikesalingam et al. 2012, 1993-2004).

If the diagnosis is delayed then patients may present with a phlegmon or appendix mass. These are generally managed conservatively with a prolonged course of antibiotics and delayed surgery in several months.

Section 5: Intussusception

Intussusception occurs when a portion of bowel telescopes into another segment, see Figure 1 below. It is the most common surgical pathology in early childhood. In children, unlike in adults, it is classically idiopathic, occurring due to enlarged intestinal lymphatic tissue, Peyer's patches, rather than a pathological lead point such as a polyp. 80-90% of presenting children are under 2 years old, however, it still can occur in those under 1 month and in older children (Mandeville, Chien, Willyerd, Mandell et al. 2012, 842-844).

Figure 1. *Diagram illustrating the process of intussusception (Remesz)*
See colour centrefold for this image.

History & Examination

The classical history is of an infant with intermittent episodes of sudden onset cramping and severe abdominal pain. The infant will often cry inconsolably and draw their legs up to the abdomen. The episodes classically occur every 15-20 minutes. The infant may vomit, progressing from non-bilious at first, to bilious later. Redcurrant jelly stool is present in approximately 50% of infants due to blood from ischaemic mucosa mixing with mucous. A palpable mass is occasionally present. This is typically sausage-shaped and felt in the right mid-abdomen, as ileocolic intussusceptions account for 90% of cases (Mandeville, Chien, Willyerd, Mandell et al. 2012, 842-844). Dance's sign, where the RIF is empty due to retraction of the caecum superiorly, is classical but uncommon.

Investigations

The infant should have basic biochemical and haematological investigations including a lactate. Patients should also have an abdominal radiograph to exclude perforation. The diagnostic investigation of choice is ultrasonography. For an experienced operator, the sensitivity and specificity approach 100%, with the classical "target sign" indicative of intussusception; see Figure 2 below (Hryhorczuk, Strouse 2009, 1975).

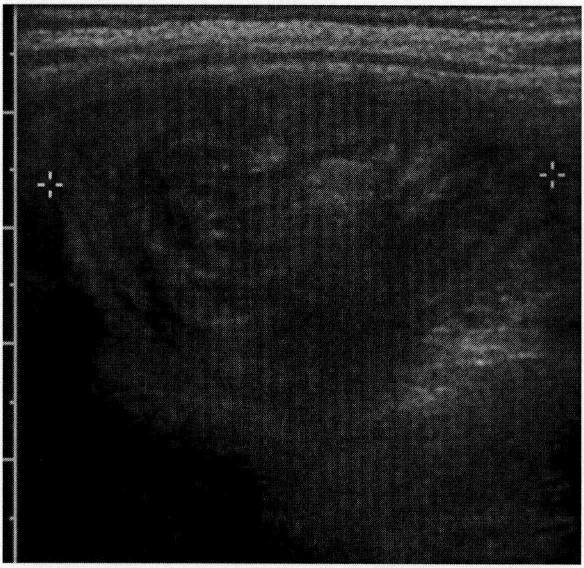

Figure 2. *Ultrasound demonstrating the classical target sign in intussusception (Gaillard)*

Management

The primary management is fluoroscopic guided reduction via hydrostatic (saline or contrast), or pneumatic (air) enema. This should only be undertaken in centres with paediatric surgery and paediatric radiology, with a haemodynamically stable child. Air enema is now typically preferred as opposed to hydrostatic enema, as it is quicker, with less radiation, and there is less peritoneal contamination if perforation occurs during the attempted reduction.

There is a possibility of perforation during enema reduction, and this can cause cardiovascular collapse due to large volume pneumoperitoneum compressing the vena cava. Therefore, the paediatric surgical team should be in attendance during the enema reduction and if there is concern for perforation during the procedure, a large bore cannula should be inserted into the abdominal cavity to reduce intra-abdominal pressure, prior to urgent surgical exploration.

In most centres, the standard protocol is a maximum of 3 attempts at enema reduction. If unsuccessful, surgical intervention is indicated, or if the infant has evidence of perforation, or is extremely unwell, surgery is the initial primary treatment. Needless to say, you will not be expected to see these children independently as the SHO. However, understanding what is required is necessary to appropriately expedite and facilitate the appropriate management. In all cases where you suspect an intussusception, Senior advice should be sought.

Typically, the child starts clear fluids post-procedure, and diet is increased as tolerated. Some centres advocate monitoring the child for 12-24 hours, as 10% will suffer a recurrence, with 50% of these within the first 72 hours.

Section 6: Neonates

As the surgical SHO, you will have less exposure to neonatal patients. However, it is important to be aware of the common conditions as you may be assisting in the management of these patients.

Obstruction

Perhaps the most urgent of presentations is the neonate with intestinal obstruction. A baby with bilious vomiting should be treated as an emergency due to the risk of structural intestinal obstruction. For such patients an abdominal radiograph should be obtained, and if suggestive of a proximal obstruction, an upper GI contrast series carried out to exclude malrotation. If distal obstruction is suspected, a contrast enema may be indicated. All these patients should have Senior led decision making, but the initial management will always include gastric decompression with a nasogastric tube on free drainage, intravenous fluid resuscitation and nil by mouth.

Malrotation

Intestinal malrotation is a congenital anomaly that occurs due to an arrest in the normal rotation of the embryonic gastrointestinal tract. The most concerning complication is that of malrotation causing mid-gut volvulus. **This is a life-threatening pathology and it is time critical.** Approximately one-third of infants with malrotation present before the age of 1 month with this complication (Fonkalsrud 2003, 477). The small bowel twists around the superior mesenteric artery, causing ischaemia to the mid gut and eventual necrosis. Infants with malrotation typically present with bilious vomiting, either because of volvulus or duodenal obstruction due to Ladd's bands crossing the duodenum.

The definitive investigation is an upper GI contrast series, which in malrotation demonstrates:

- Duodeno-jejunal (DJ) junction on the right side of the abdomen
- DJ junction lying inferior to the duodenal bulb
- Second and third parts of duodenal not lying in the retroperitoneum

This should only be performed in stable infants. If a child has bilious vomiting with distension and peritonism – urgent surgery is required as this is time critical and investigations are unnecessary.

Operative correction of malrotation is known as a Ladd's procedure, whereby any congenital adhesions (Ladd's bands) are divided and the mesenteric base widened to reduce the risk of future volvulus.

Hirschsprung disease

Hirschsprung disease is a congenital disorder of the gut, whereby there is an absence of ganglion cells in the myenteric and submucosal plexus. It typically affects the recto-sigmoid region; however, it can also affect larger sections of colon and in rare cases can be pan-intestinal. There is an association with Trisomy 21. Due to the lack of ganglion cells, the affected bowel is persistently contracted and cannot relax. This causes a functional bowel obstruction.

The majority of patients will be diagnosed in the neonatal period and will classically have failed to pass meconium within 48 hours of birth. They may have abdominal distension, vomiting and an explosive expulsion of gas and stool on digital rectal examination.

Patients should be managed as per bowel obstruction, in addition to broad spectrum antibiotics and twice daily rectal washouts. In the United Kingdom, the standard diagnostic test is a rectal suction biopsy, in addition to a contrast enema.

Surgery is required for these patients. Traditionally, these patients had a defunctioning stoma after diagnosis, and definitive surgery planned for a later date. However, surgery can now be performed in one stage, and the patients can be decompressed with rectal washouts until surgery is required. There is a risk of Hirschsprung associated enterocolitis in both pre-operative and post-operative patients, and this can be a severe and potentially fatal complication that requires prompt medical management with fluid resuscitation, broad-spectrum antibiotics and intestinal decompression.

Necrotising enterocolitis

Neonates with necrotising enterocolitis (NEC) are typically under the neonatal team with surgical input as requested by the neonatal doctors. This is one of the most common neonatal surgical emergencies and is characterised by ischaemic necrosis of the intestine. It is much more common in pre-term neonates. If suspected, patients should have a plain abdominal radiograph. Features suggestive of NEC include dilated or thick-walled bowel loops, or bowel wall pneumatosis, shown in Figure 3 below.

The management is typically nil by mouth, gastric decompression and broad-spectrum antibiotics. This is in combination with serial abdominal examinations, repeat blood tests and imaging. Medical management is instigated for 5 – 10 days, and surgical intervention indicated with clinical deterioration on maximal medical management, or in the presence of pneumoperitoneum. Operative management should also be considered when there are multiple relative indications, such as X-ray findings of:

portal venous air, a persistent fixed bowel loop, pneumatosis, or a worsening clinical picture. It is difficult to make this decision based on one assessment, and multiple examinations are typically required.

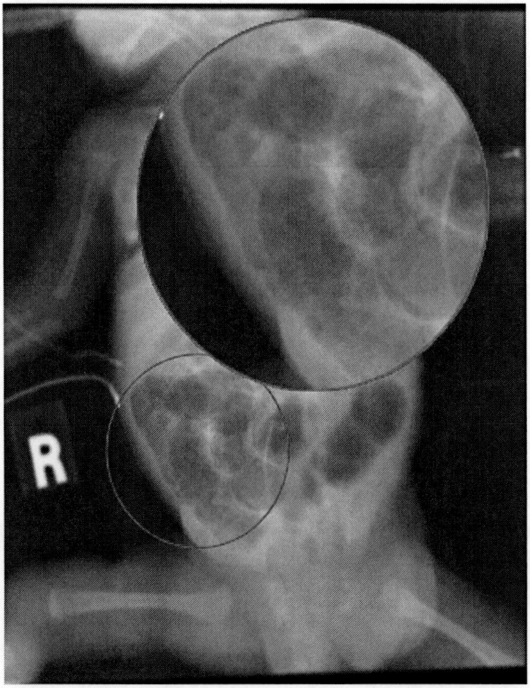

Figure 3. *Intestinal pneumatosis in a child with NEC (Rads)*

Tracheo-oesophageal fistula

Tracheo-oesophageal fistula (TOF), with associated oesophageal atresia, is an uncommon but important condition in neonatal surgical units. Occasionally the infants will have an antenatal diagnosis, with polyhydramnios and an absent stomach bubble identified on obstetric ultrasound scans. The clinical presentation depends on the exact nature of the anomaly, but with a combined TOF and oesophageal atresia (OA), the infant will typically present with drooling, choking and respiratory distress, and an inability to feed. A diagnosis of oesophageal atresia is made after a nasogastric tube is unable to be inserted. Typically, it will only pass 10-15cm, and on radiograph, will be seen curled in the upper oesophageal pouch: Figure 4.

Surgical intervention is mandated although the approach and timing depend on the nature of the anomaly and the co-morbidities of the infant.

Section 7: Practical skills

Feeding Tubes

As the SHO on call, you may occasionally be asked to see children with issues with their feeding tubes. There are a variety of feeding tubes, with multiple different types of each. They can be arranged by location:

Gastric tubes are placed into the stomach, and are used for patients with structural abnormalities or with swallowing difficulties. There are two main forms – standard gastrostomy tubes which have a long external tube and low-profile gastrostomy devices, also known as "buttons". Button devices have the advantage of less external components, but are not typically placed primarily, thus children will often have a standard gastrostomy tube swapped to a button device at a later date.

Gastrojejunostomy (GJ) tubes are tubes inserted via gastrostomy but with a much longer internal tube. These allow for jejunal feeding and the ability to perform gastric decompression. These are placed either endoscopically, or under fluoroscopic guidance by interventional radiology.

Jejunostomy tubes are tubes that enter the jejunum directly to allow jejunal feeding. They are initially placed surgically, either via an open, or laparoscopic technique. As the small bowel is not meant for large boluses, any infants fed via a jejunal tube require continuous, as opposed to bolus feeds.

Tube care

Standard gastrostomy tubes should be rotated 360 degrees and advanced 2-3cm into the stomach and pulled back to the original position on at least a weekly basis to prevent buried bumper syndrome. Low profile gastrostomy tubes should be rotated through 90-180 degrees daily, to prevent adherence of the balloon to the stomach wall and the water in the balloon should be changed weekly. **Rotation should not be done for tubes with a jejunal extension as this can easily lead to misplacement**. All tubes should be flushed before and after feeds, and before and after medications. Tubes should not be removed within 6-8 weeks after placement, as the tract will not be well developed.

If a gastrostomy tube is inadvertently removed, some form of replacement tube should be placed **within 4 hours** as the tract will otherwise close. In the acute post-operative period, this should be replaced with a Foley catheter – and you should select the largest size that fits. If it is a mature tract, then either the same tube, or a replacement device should be sited. In such cases, correct re-insertion needs to be confirmed under fluoroscopic guidance.

Intravenous access

For those new to paediatrics, the placement of peripheral cannulae and blood taking can be both daunting and stressful. In paediatric patients, preparation is key. One must ensure that all efforts are made to make the child as comfortable as possible. This includes the presence of parents, **additional support from nursing staff and play preparation**. In day-time hours, play specialists can assist, especially for children with difficult access and/or multiple previous cannulation attempts. It should be performed in a clinical treatment room, trying to avoid the child's bed space if possible. You should avoid the arm that the child prefers and try to avoid cannulating near joints. Local anaesthetic creams should be utilised. Sucrose solution can be used in infants under 3 months of age, via the buccal route, or a dummy dipped into the solution. However, this should be prescribed, and you must consult guidelines regarding the frequency and dosage.

Local anaesthetic

Ametop (tetracaine) and EMLA (lidocaine and prilocaine) are the most commonly used topical anaesthetics. Ametop is licensed for those over 1 month of age, and EMLA for those over 1 year old. Ametop should be applied for 30-45 minutes, and not for any longer, whereas EMLA requires at least an hour to take effect. Sterile dressings or clingfilm can be applied over the cream to secure it in place. Ametop typically dilates blood vessels, whereas EMLA cream constricts. In those over 5 years old, ethyl chloride ("cold spray"), can also be utilised. It has no anaesthetic properties but acts as a vapo-coolant. After application, the needle should be inserted within 30 seconds before the effect wears off.

Blood sampling

For blood taking, standard venepuncture, with consideration of the above guidelines, can be used in older children. In infants, a blood draw can be performed via either a heel-prick or finger-prick. The same supportive environment as outlined above, should be adopted in this scenario. A heel-prick is suitable for those under 6 months, whereas a finger prick is more suitable in those over 6 months of age. For a heel-prick, the lancet should be used at either the lateral or the medial plantar surface. For a finger-prick, you should take it from the side of the ball of the finger, perpendicular to the lines of the fingerprint. This should ideally be taken from either the second or third finger.

Section 8: Prescribing

As an SHO on call, prescribing can be intimidating for those unfamiliar with paediatrics. Medications should be prescribed with strict accordance with national and local guidelines. Fluid prescribing needs care and attention, and there are two forms of prescriptions – maintenance fluids and dehydration fluids. You must, therefore, consider the child's current degree of dehydration, their ongoing losses and maintenance fluid requirements. Urine output should be >1ml/kg/hr in those over 2 years old, and >2ml/kg/hr in those under 2. Children on prolonged intravenous fluids should have accurate input/output monitoring, in addition to daily weights and daily electrolytes. Unlike adults, paediatric fluids typically come in 500ml bags.

In children, maintenance fluids can be calculated over 24 hours and then divided to give an hourly rate. A calculation for this is relatively simple to follow:

- 100ml/kg/24hrs for the first 10kg
- 50ml/kg/24hrs for the subsequent 10kg
- 20ml/kg/24hrs for any additional bodyweight above 20kg

In children, electrolyte requirements are 2-4mmol/kg/24hrs of sodium and 1-2mmol/kg/24 hrs of potassium. To meet these requirements for maintenance fluids, a prescription of 500ml of 0.9% saline + 5% dextrose with 10mmol KCL will be sufficient for most patients. However, at all times, seek Senior support if uncertain. In critically unwell patients with a significant fluid deficit, a fluid bolus of 10-20ml/kg of 0.9% saline can be used to partially correct dehydration. If a child remains unstable after

40ml/kg of fluid boluses, expert advice should be sought from paediatric intensive care.

Neonatal Fluids

This rule does not apply for neonates. In neonates the fluid requirements are 60ml/kg/day on day 1, followed by 90ml/kg/24hrs on day 2, 120ml/kg/24hrs on day 3 and 150ml/kg/24hrs thereafter. Small for size, or premature, infants require more fluids, typically an extra 20ml/kg/24 hrs for those under 1.5kg and 40ml/kg/24hrs in those under 1kg. Electrolyte requirements are extremely important in neonates and need to be added to the bag manually.

Conclusion

Paediatric surgery is a rewarding yet demanding specialty and for those cross-covering, Senior advice should be sought for decision making. It is a Senior led specialty and an SHO should not feel worried about asking for help with even the simplest of tasks.

References

Appendicitis in the young child: a continuing diagnostic challenge. Nance ML, Adamson WT, Hedrick HL. Pediatr Emerg Care. 2000;16(3):160.

Current concepts in inguinal hernia in infants and children. Grosfeld JL. World J Surg. 1989;13(5):506.

Diagnosing pediatric appendicitis: usefulness of laboratory markers. Kwan KY, Nager AL. Am J Emerg Med. 2010 Nov;28(9):1009-15. Epub 2010 Mar 9.

Epidemiology of inguinal hernia in preterm neonates. Peevy KJ, Speed FA, Hoff CJ. Pediatrics. 1986;77(2):246.

Fonkalsrud E. Rotational anomalies and volvulus. In: Principles of Pediatric Surgery, O'Neill JA et al (Ed), Mosby, St. Louis 2003. p.477.

Gaillard F, [GFDL 1.3CC BY-SA 3.0, GFDL 1.3 (www.gnu.org/licenses/fdl-1.3.html) or CC BY-SA 3.0 (https://creativecommons.org/licenses/by-sa/3.0)], https://commons.wikimedia.org/wiki/File:Intussusception_on_ultrasound.jpg - via Wikimedia Commons. Last accessed 09/12/19

Impact of surgical approach on outcome in 622 consecutive pyloromyotomies at a pediatric teaching institution. Perger L, Fuchs JR, Komidar L Mooney DP. J Pediatr Surg. 2009;44(11):2119.

Importance of diarrhea as a presenting symptom of appendicitis in very young children. Horwitz JR, Gursoy M, Jaksic T, Lally KP. Am J Surg. 1997;173(2):80.

Inguinal hernia in infants: the fate of the testis following incarceration. Puri P, Guiney EJ, O'Donnell B. J Pediatr Surg. 1984;19(1):44.

Intussusception: clinical presentations and imaging characteristics. Mandeville K, Chien M, Willyerd FA, Mandell G, Hostetler MA, Bulloch B. Pediatr Emerg Care. 2012 Sep;28(9):842-4.

Laparoscopic pyloromyotomy. Downey EC Jr. Semin Pediatr Surg. 1998;7(4):220.

Laparoscopic versus open appendectomy for complicated and uncomplicated appendicitis in children. Markar SR, Blackburn S, Cobb R, Karthikesalingam A, Evans J, Kinross J, Faiz O. J Gastrointest Surg. 2012 Oct;16(10):1993-2004. Epub 2012 Jul 19.

Management of paediatric hernia. Bowling K, Hart N, Cox P, Srinivas G. BMJ. 2017;359:j4484

Neonatal acute appendicitis: a proposed algorithm for timely diagnosis. Schwartz KL, Gilad E, Sigalet D, Yu W, Wong AL. J Pediatr Surg. 2011 Nov;46(11):2060-4.

Pyloric muscle in asymptomatic infants: sonographic evaluation and discrimination from idiopathic hypertrophic pyloric stenosis. Rohrschneider WK, Mittnacht H, Darge K. Pediatr Radiol. 1998 Jun; 28(6):429-34.

Rads [CC BY-SA 3.0 (https://creativecommons.org/licenses/by-sa/3.0) or CC BY-SA 3.0 (https://creativecommons.org/licenses/by-sa/3.0)], https://en.wikipedia.org/wiki/Necrotizing_enterocolitis#/media/File:Necrotizing_enterocolitis_202.jpg via Wikimedia Commons

Remesz O. https://en.wikipedia.org/wiki/Intussusception_(medical_disorder)#/media/File:Intussusception_EN.svg. Creative commons licence held at: https://creativecommons.org/licenses/by-sa/3.0, from Wikimedia Commons, last accessed 20/01/19

The epidemiology of appendicitis and appendectomy in the United States. Addiss DG, Shaffer N, Fowler BS, Tauxe, RV. Am J Epidemiol. 1990;132(5):910.

The presentation of appendicitis in preadolescent children. Colvin JM, Bachur R, Kharbanda A. Pediatr Emerg Care. 2007 Dec;23(12):849-55.

Validation of US as a first-line diagnostic test for assessment of pediatric ileocolic intussusception. Hryhorczuk AL, Strouse PJ. Pediatr Radiol. 2009;39(10):1075. Epub 2009 Aug 6

Chapter 1: Breast Surgery

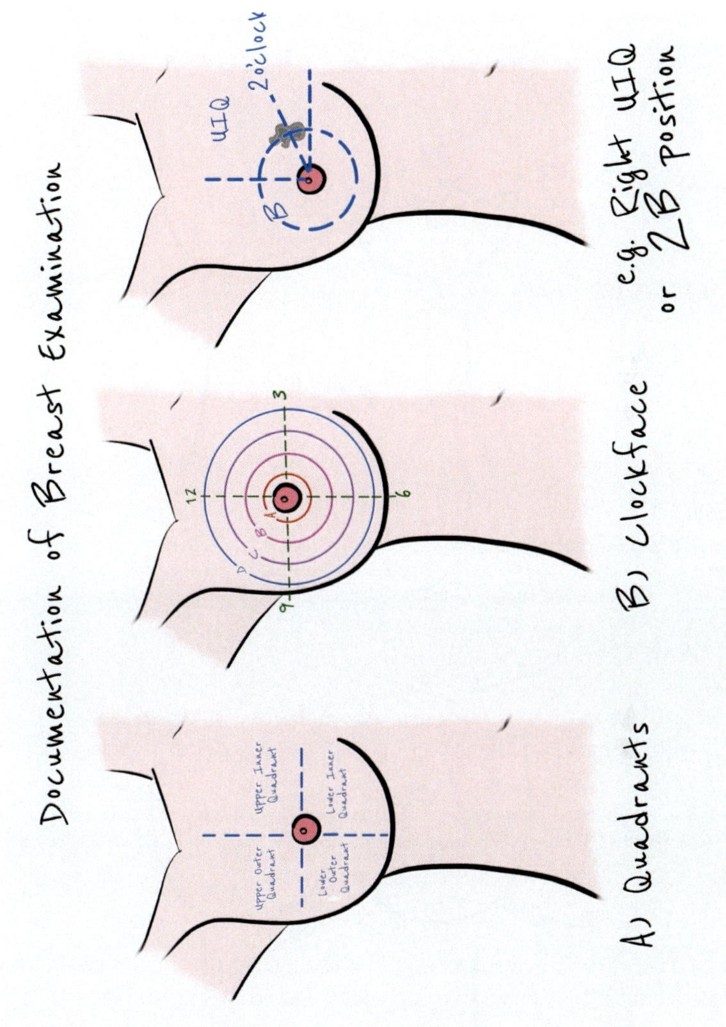

Figure 1. *Diagram of documenting in clock-face and quadrants*

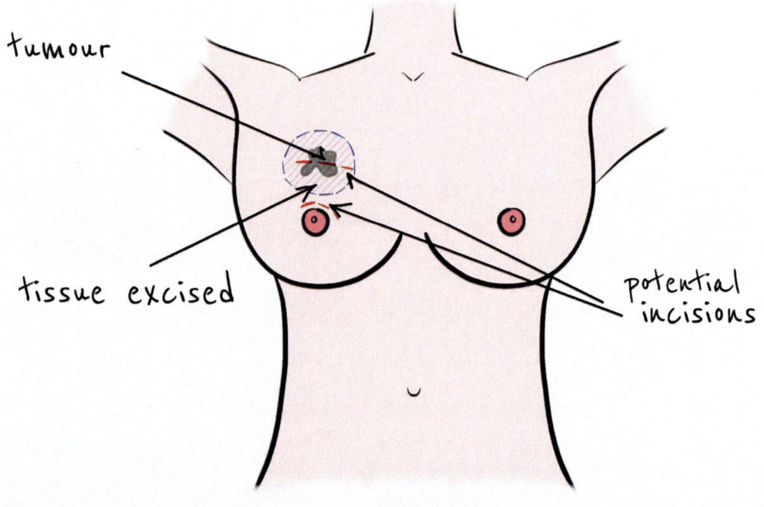

Figure 2. *Wide local excision*

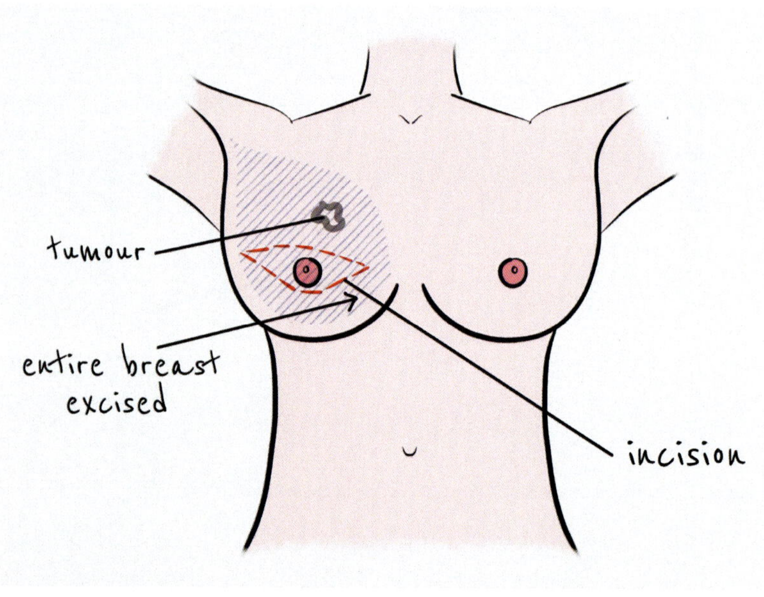

Figure 3. *Mastectomy*

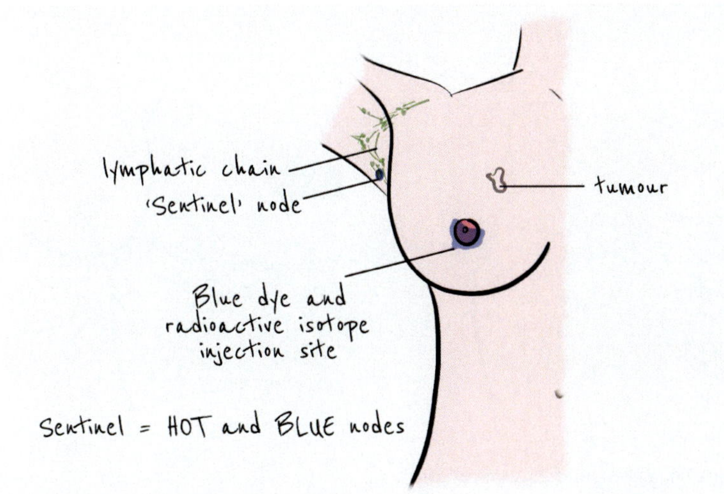

Figure 4. *Sentinel lymph node biopsy*

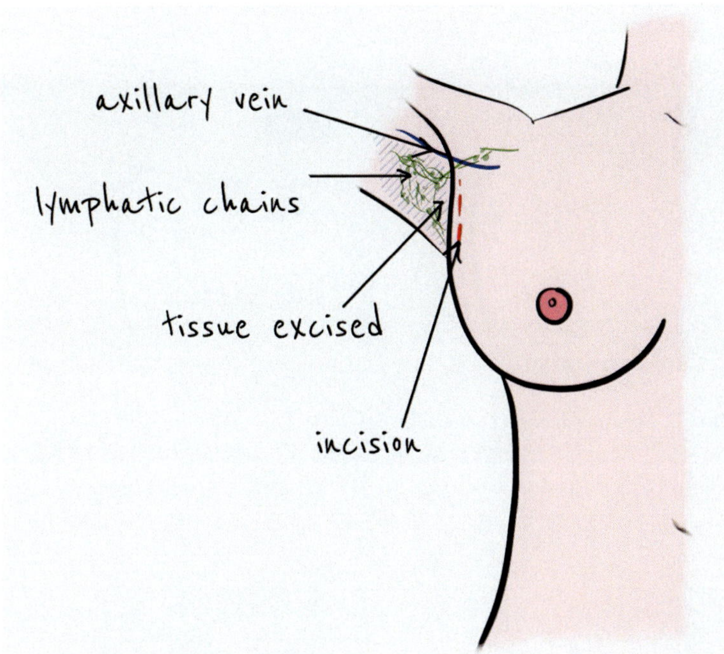

Figure 5. *Axillary lymph node biopsy*

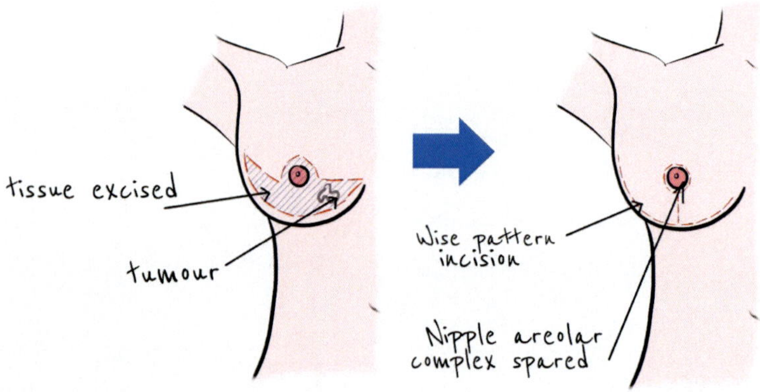

Figure 6. *Therapeutic mammoplasty*

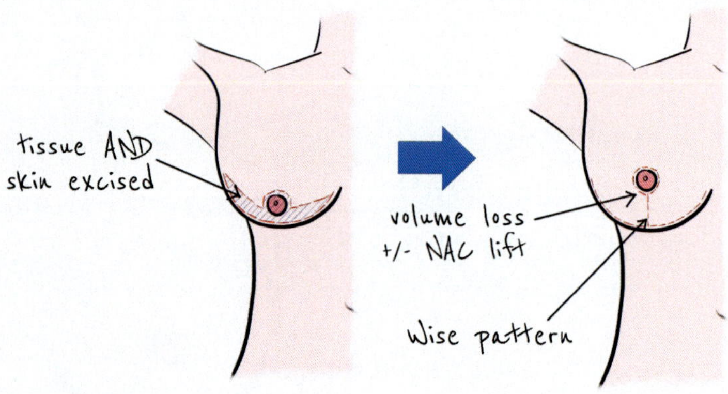

Figure 7. *Breast reduction (symmetrising)*

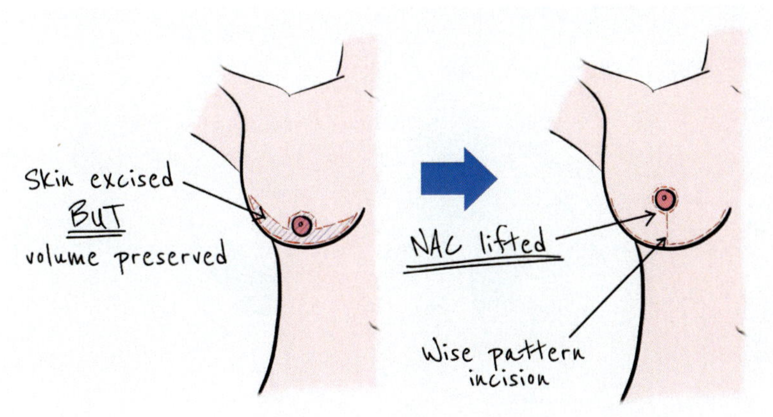

Figure 8. *Mastopexy (symmetrising)*

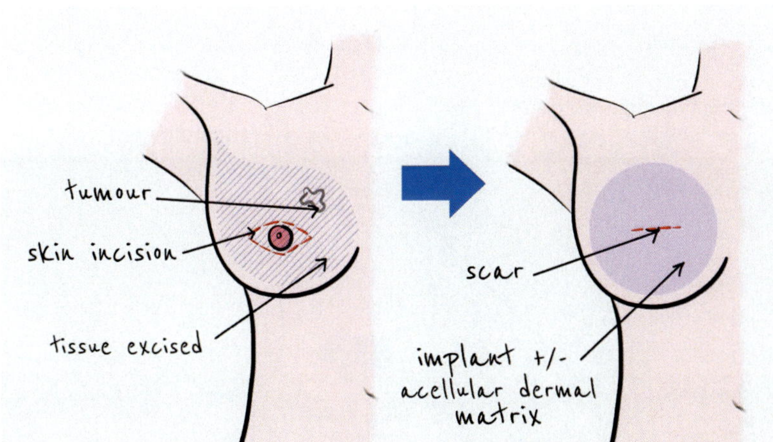

Figure 9. *Implant based reconstruction +/- acellular dermal matrix*

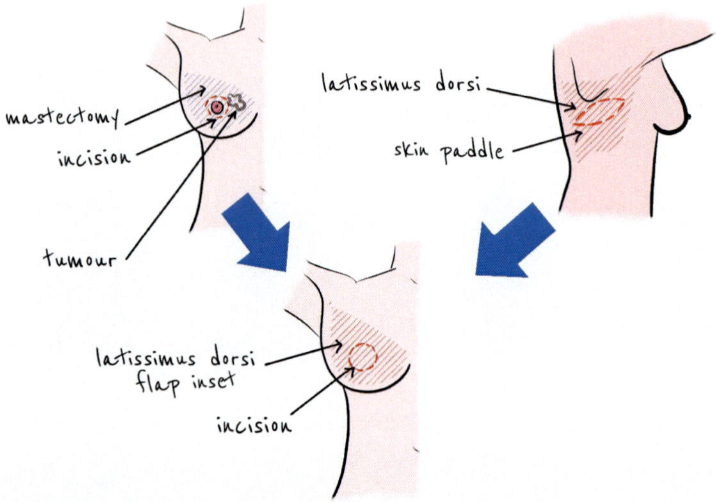

Figure 10. *Latissimus dorsi*

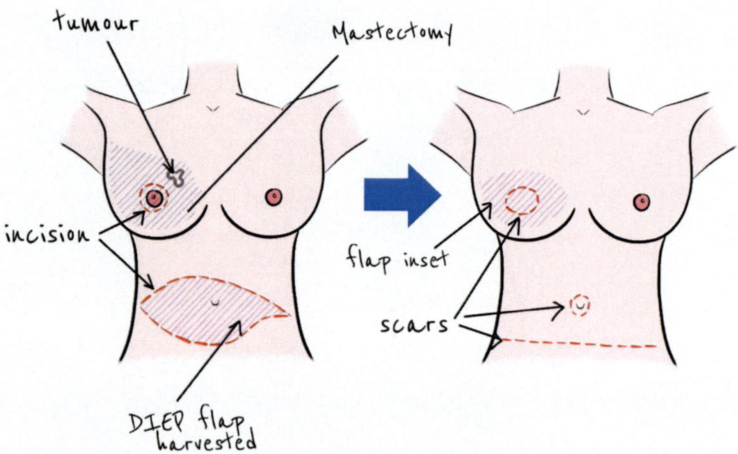

Figure 11. *Deep inferior epigastric artery reconstruction*

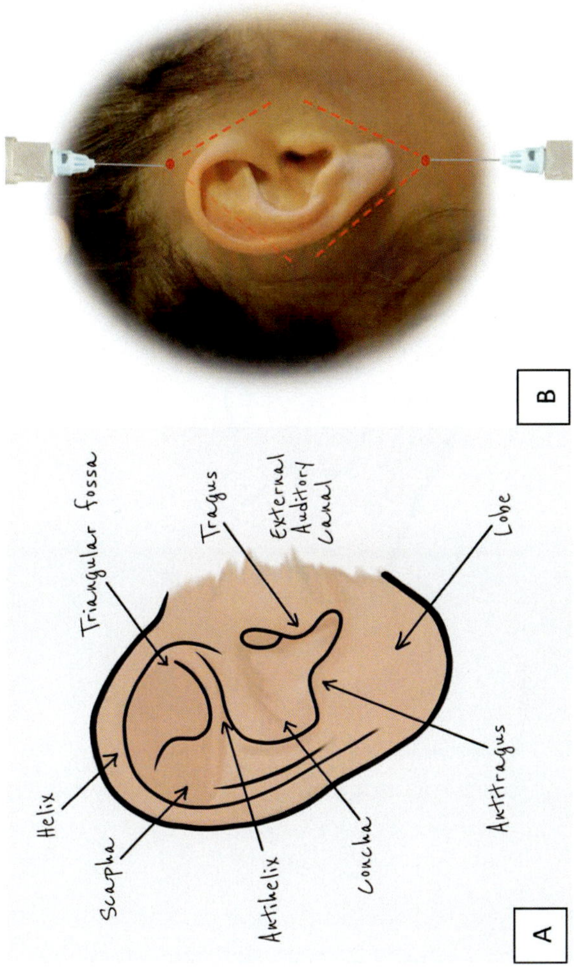

Inject:
1. At the junction of the superior helix and scalp– infero-anteriorly and infero-posteriorly to the ear
2. Just inferior to the junction of the lobule and face– supero-anteriorly and supero-posterior to the ear

Figure 14. *A) Normal ear anatomy B) Pinna block*

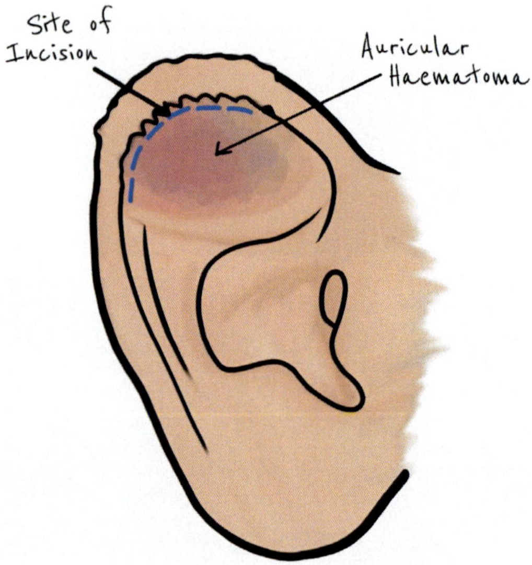

Figure 15. *Incision of pinna haematoma*

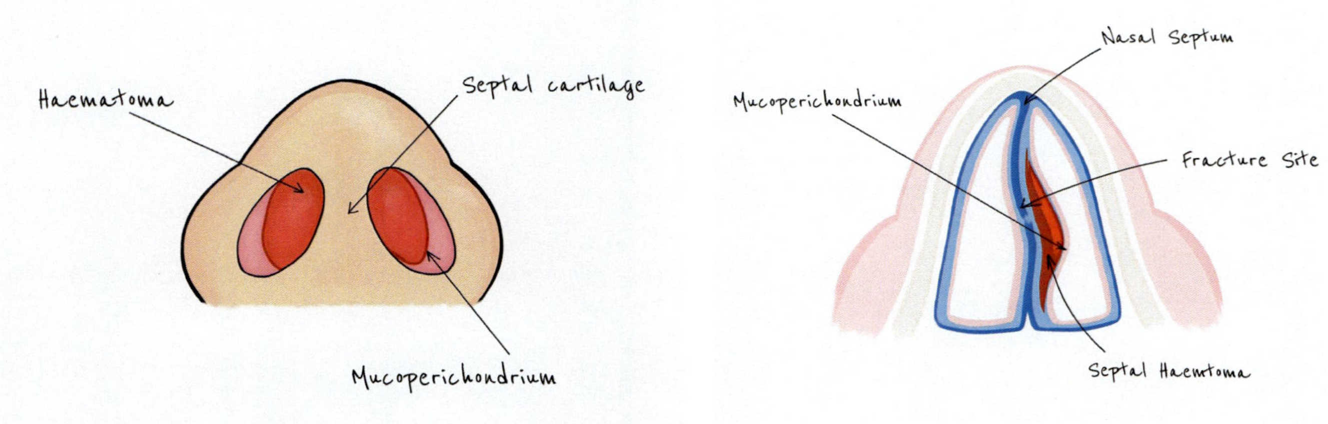

Figure 20. *Septal haematoma*

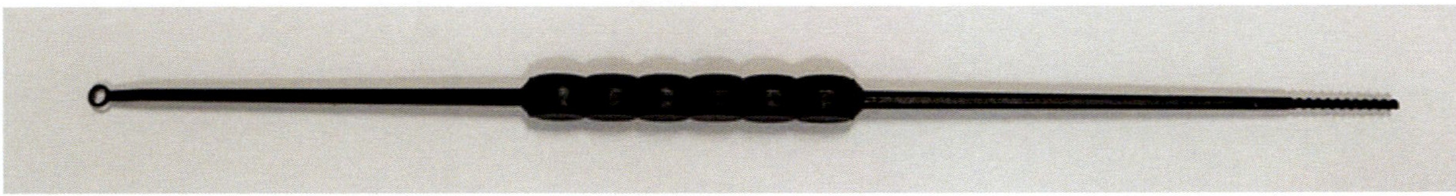

Figure 22. *Jobson Horne Probe*

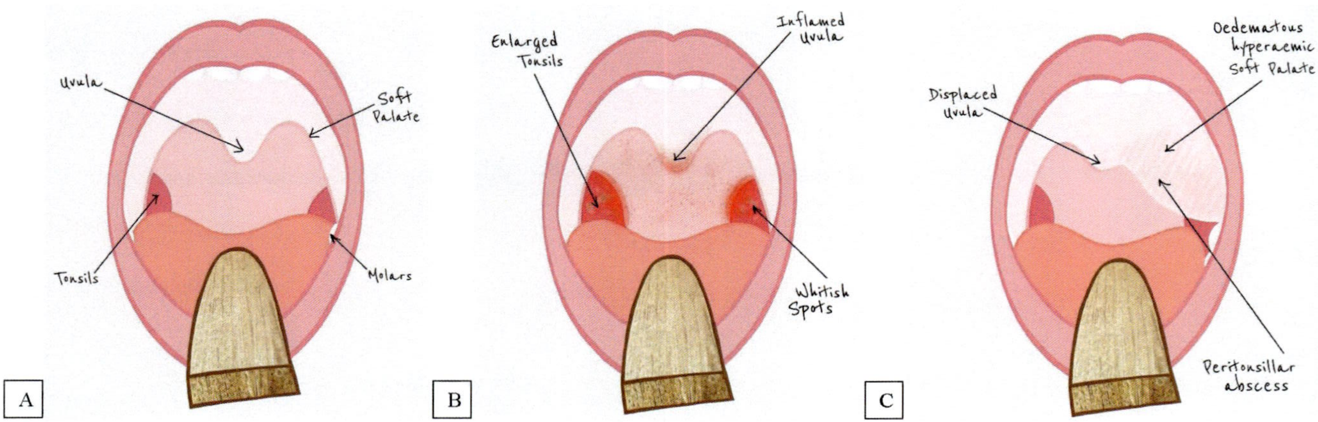

Figure 25. *A) Normal Oropharynx B) Tonsilitis C) Peritonsillar abscess*

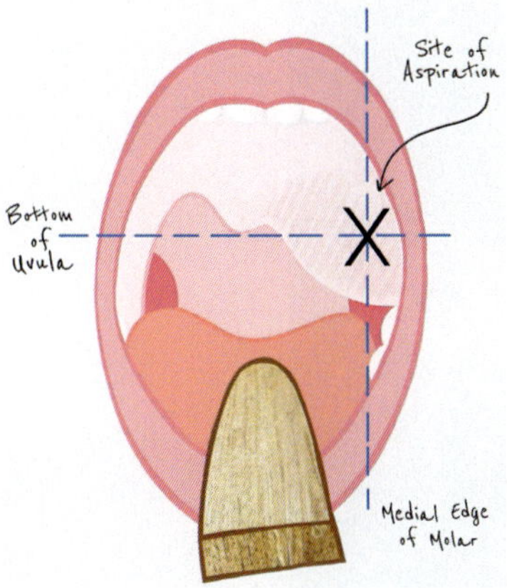

Aspiration of peritonsillar abscess

- Ask someone to show you how to perform this the first time
- Explain the procedure to the patient, including that there will be some bleeding and possibly a foul taste in the mouth
- Sit the patient up with their head rested against the bed, spray the throat with topical anaesthetic such as xylocaine spray (ask them to keep it in their throat and then spit out)
- Prepare your equipment (white needle, 10ml syringe, metal tongue depressor, sick bowl, tissues, suction, head torch)
- Some people create a guard for the needle to prevent it going too deep by cutting 1cm off the end of a needle sheath and replacing it over the needle
- Wear a head torch and with the tongue depressor in your non-dominant hand, insert the needle into the most prominent/fluctuant part of the abscess and draw back on the syringe until there is no further pus
- OR aspirate at a point where a horizontal line traced from the base of the uvula intersects a vertical line traced from the medial aspect of the lower molar teeth
- If aspiration fails initially, further attempts slightly superomedially and inferolaterally to the first point may be tried with the patients consent
- Be aware that the internal carotid artery lies posterior and lateral to the tonsillar pillar

Figure 26. *Peritonsillar abscess drainage*

Chapter 3: General Surgery

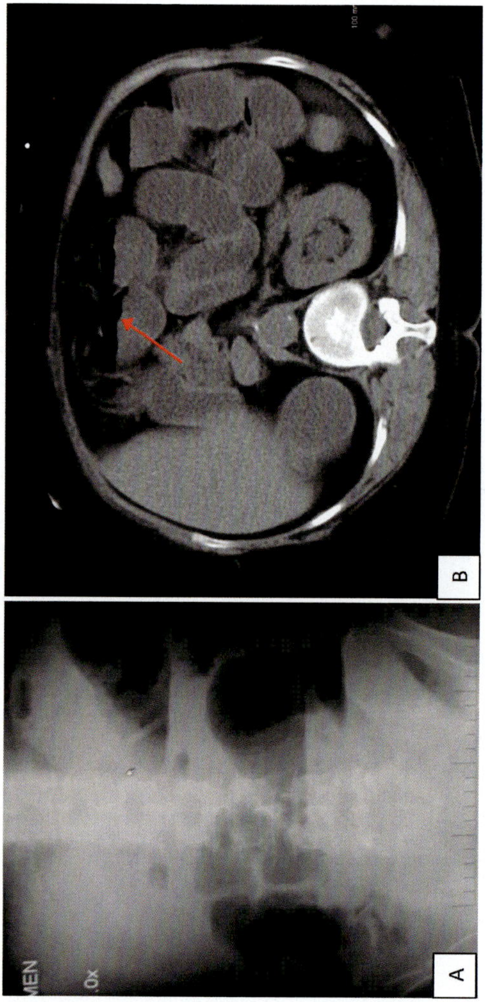

Figure 1: *A) Abdominal radiograph demonstrating small bowel obstruction (*Heilman 1a, n.d*); B) Axial image of a computerised tomography scan demonstrating small bowel obstruction. The red arrow indicates the air/fluid level typical of bowel obstruction (*Heilman 1b).

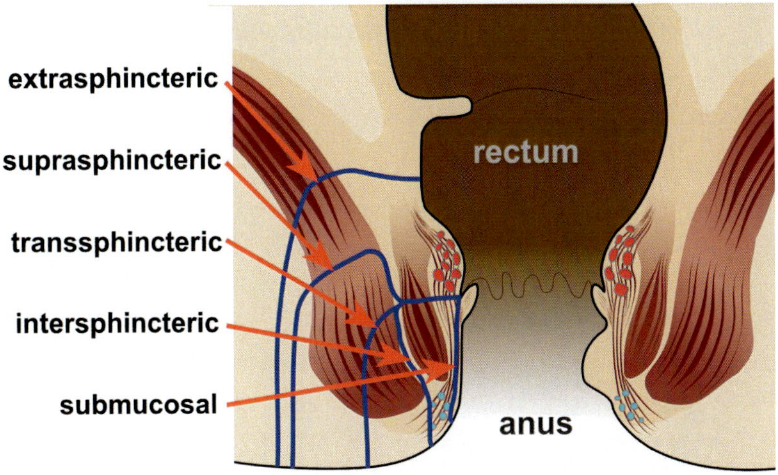

Figure 6: *Types of perianal fistulae based on their location in relation to the anal sphincters (Mcort)*

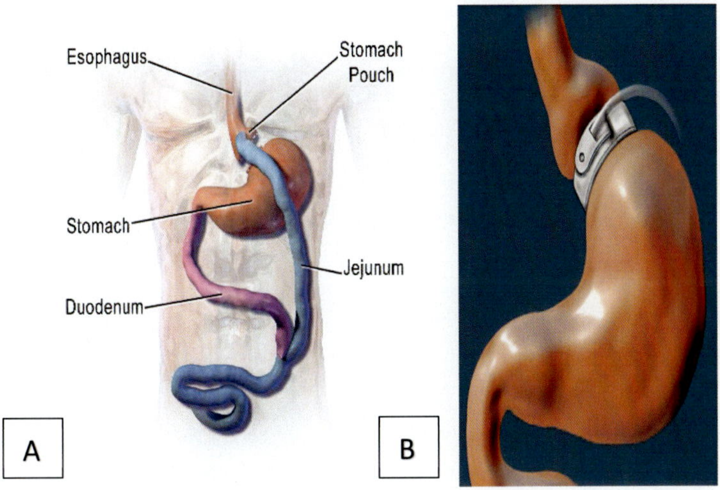

Figure 7: *Images demonstrating A) Roux-en-Y gastric bypass (Blaus); B) adjustable gastric band (Xopusmagnumx)*

Chapter 4: Oral and Maxillofacial Surgery

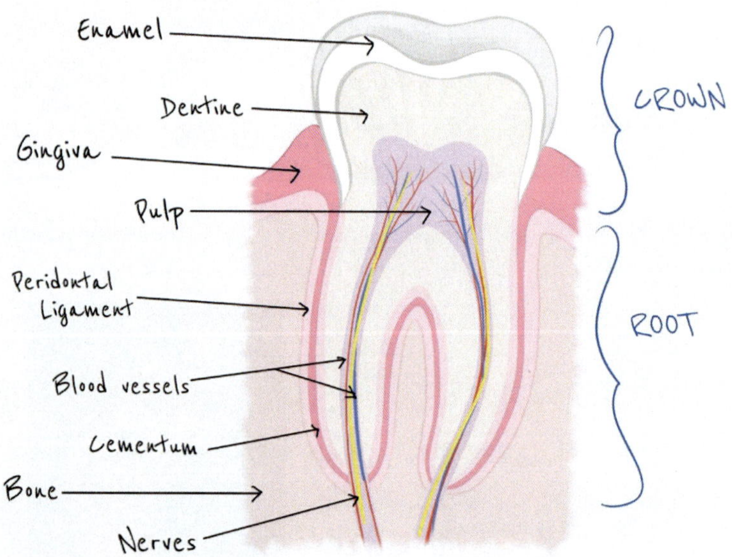

Figure 2. *Simplified tooth anatomy*

Chapter 5: Paediatric Surgery

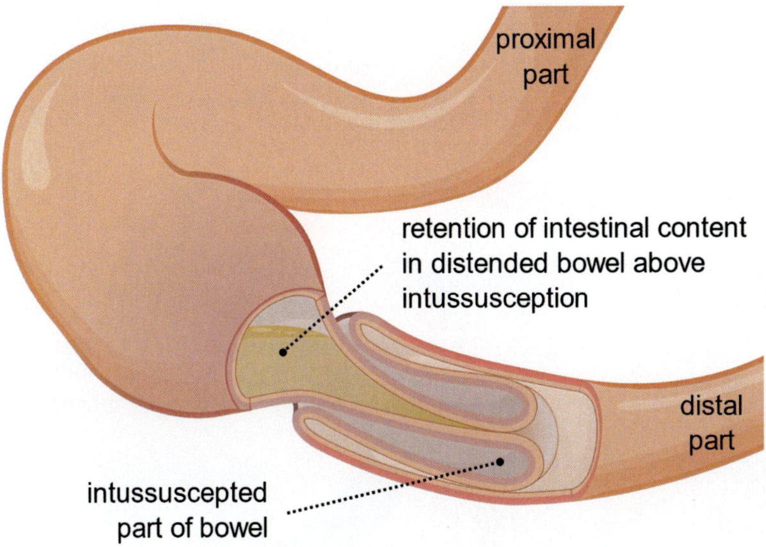

Figure 1. *Diagram illustrating the process of intussusception (Remesz, n.y)*

Chapter 6: Plastic Surgery

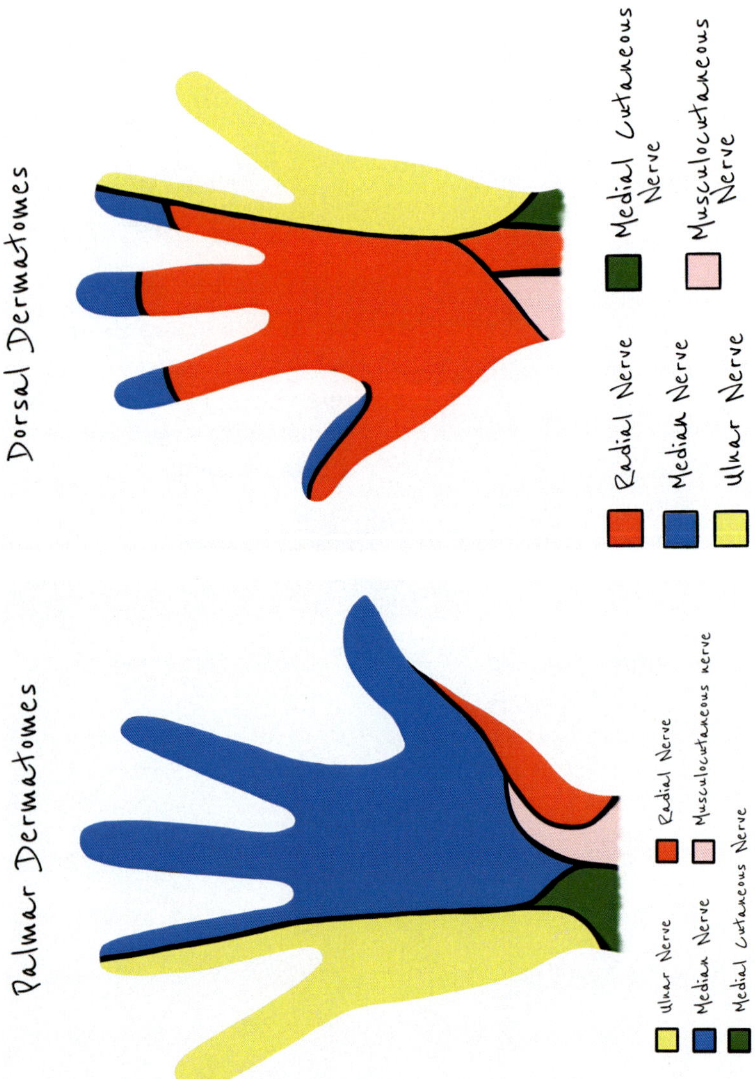

Figure 1. *Hand and forearm dermatomes (Palmar and Dorsal)*

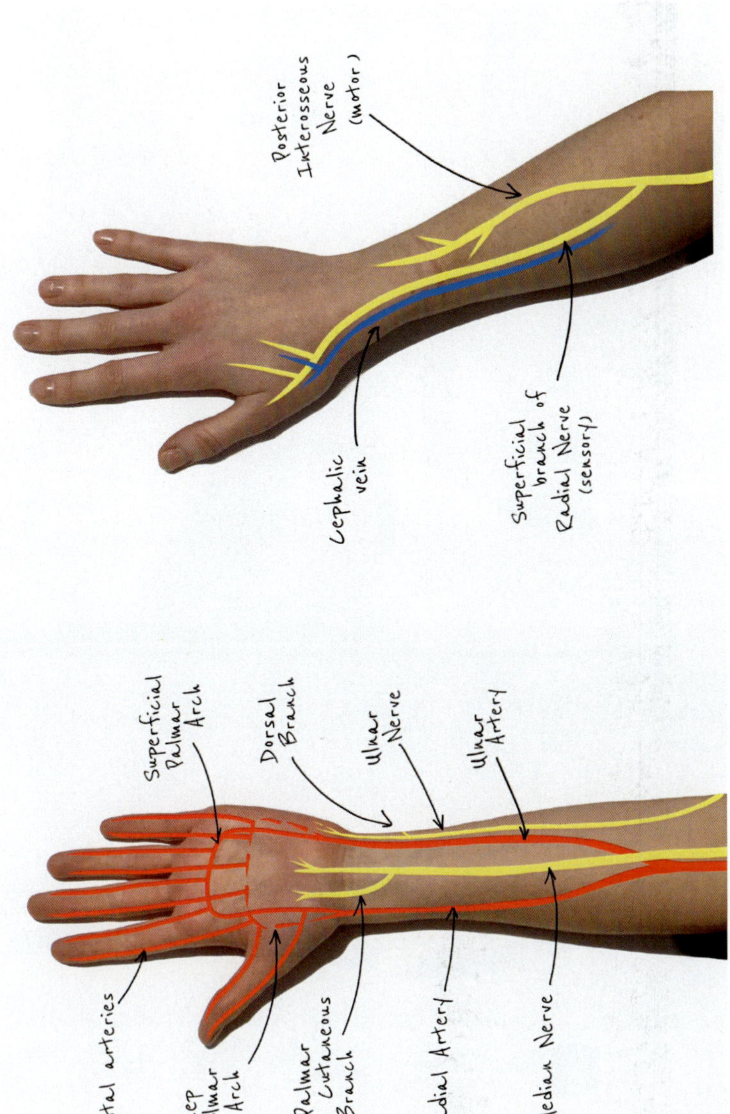

Figure 2. *Major forearm nerves and arteries*

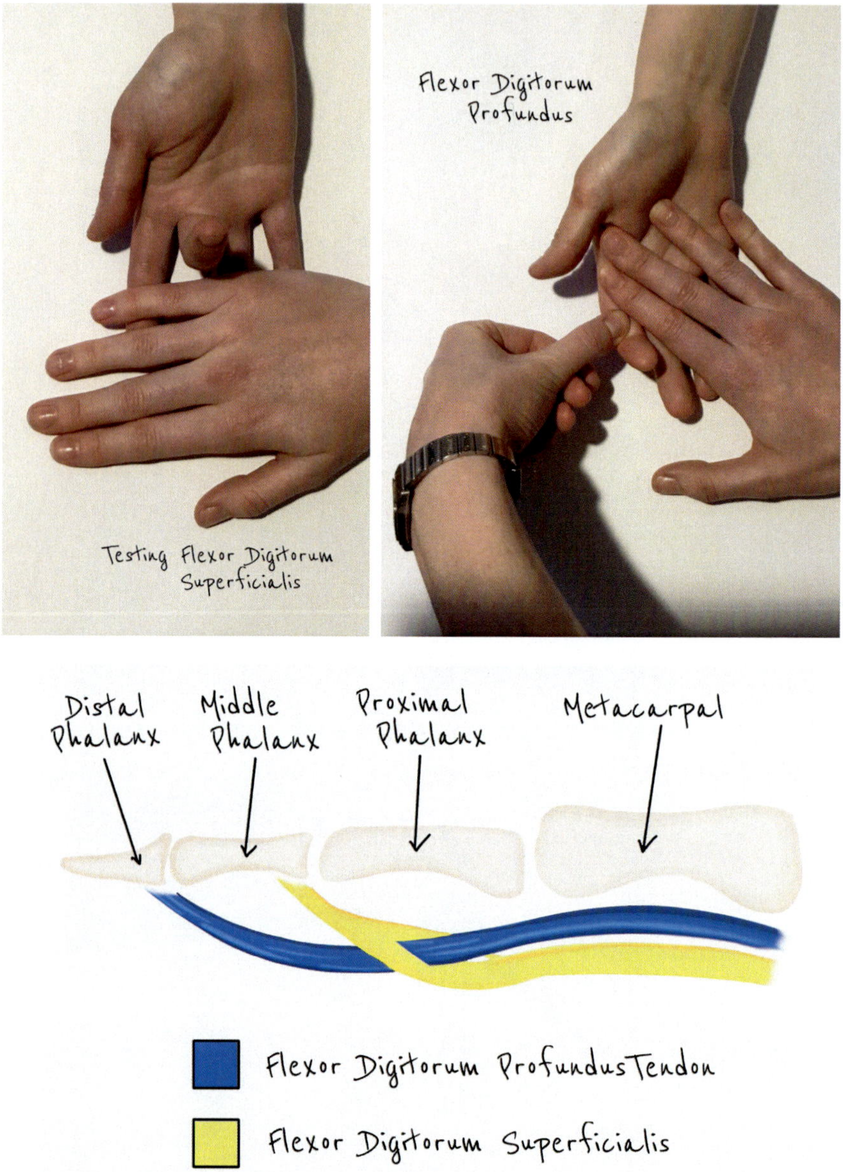

Figure 3. *FDP and FDS anatomy and examination*

SUPERFICIAL/ ERYTHEMA		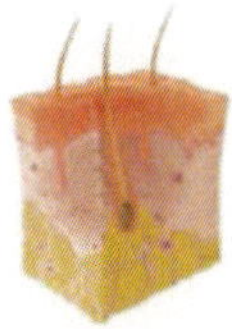	☑ Involves epidermis only ☑ Red ☑ Brisk capillary refill ☑ Skin is dry and intact ☑ No blisters ☑ Painful ☑ Erythema not included in %TBSA ☑ Heals within 3-7 days with analgesia & application of non-perfumed moisturiser	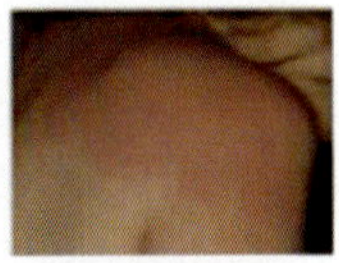
SUPERFICIAL PARTIAL THICKNESS		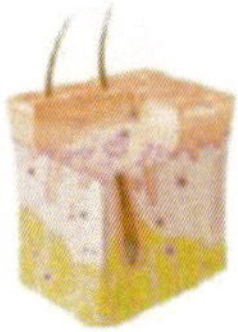	☑ Pale pink/red ☑ Brisk capillary refill ☑ Exudate present ☑ Intact or collapsed blisters may be present ☑ Painful ☑ Should heal within 14-21 days with non-adherent & absorbent dressings ☑ Refer to **Blister Management Guideline** ☑ Refer to **local Burn Service** if >3% (adults) & >1% (children)	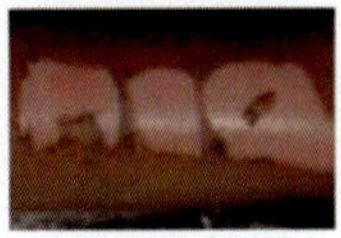
DEEP DERMAL		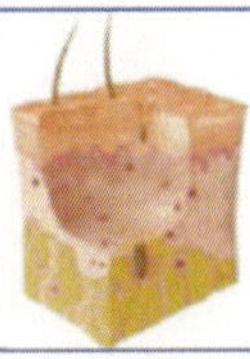	☑ Dark pink/red or white ☑ Mottled, stained, cherry red ☑ Delayed or absent capillary refill ☑ Dull/variable sensation ☑ Surgical intervention may be required ☑ Circumferential burns need urgent discussion ☑ Refer to **local Burn Service**	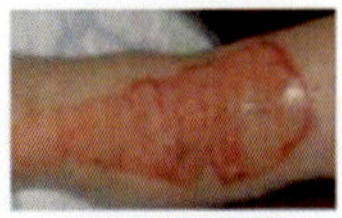
FULL THICKNESS		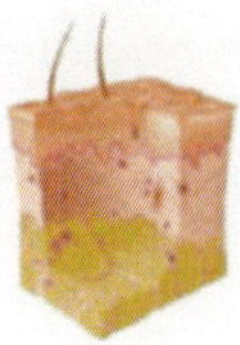	☑ White, black, brown or yellow ☑ Dry and leathery ☑ Thrombosed vessels may be visible ☑ Eschar may be present ☑ No capillary refill ☑ No sensation ☑ Surgical intervention & long term scar management required ☑ Circumferential burns need urgent discussion ☑ Refer to **local Burn Service**	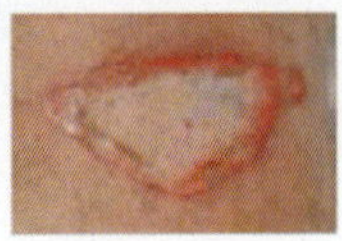

Figure 4. *Assessment of burn depth – Taken from the LSEBN Burn Depth Assessment Guidance* (LSEBN 2015a)

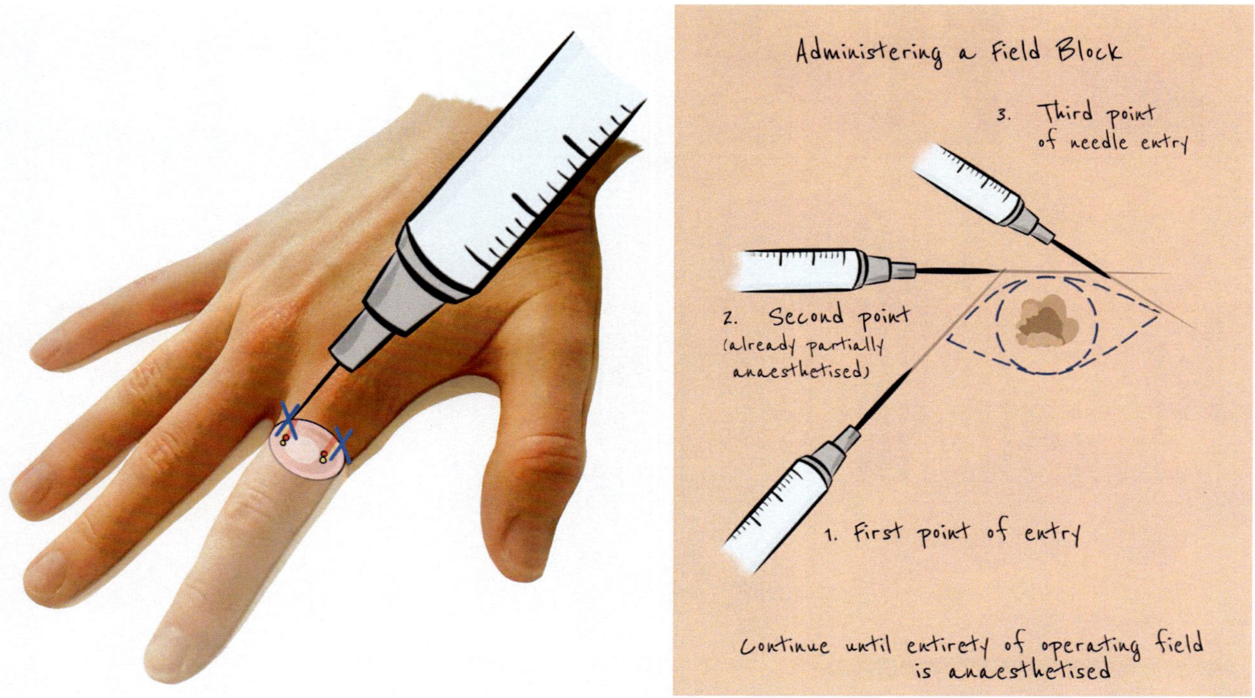

Figure 5. *Left image: Ring block: Inject bilaterally as shown with the 'X'. Also infiltrate into the subcutaneous tissue between the 'X' on the dorsum of the finger. Right image: Field block technique.*

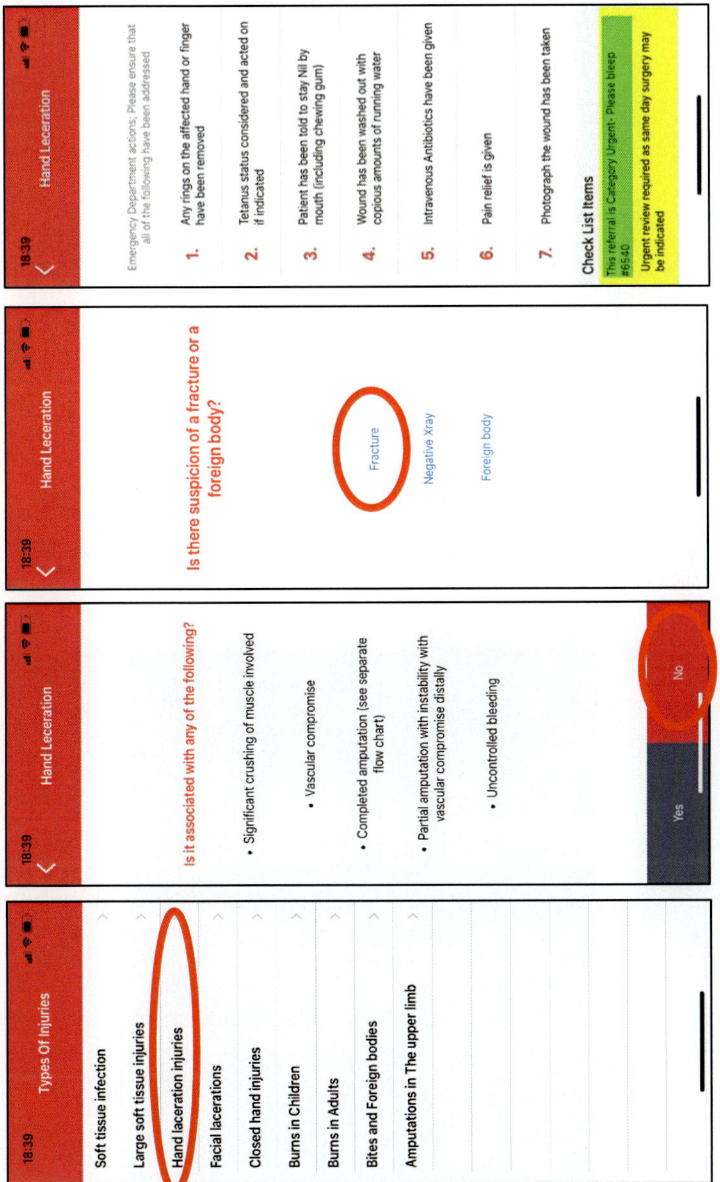

Figure 7. HIPE app interface with example of pathway for hand laceration injuries (left to right). Selected options highlighted in red.

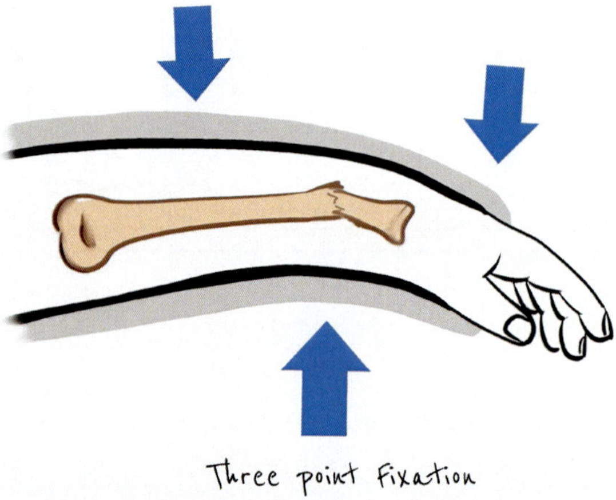

Figure 2. *Locations for 3-point fixation in a wrist fracture. Note how the intact periosteal hinge acts to align the fracture.*

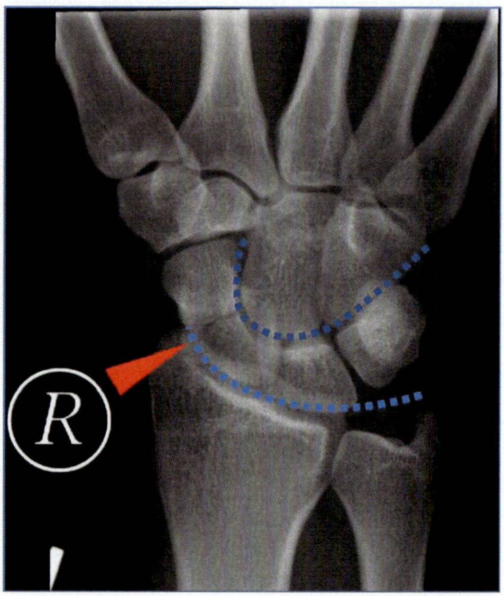

Figure 3. *Gilulas ARCS in blue on an AP radiograph of the wrist. The red arrow points to a scaphoid waist fracture. 1 (Wikipedia, 2019)*

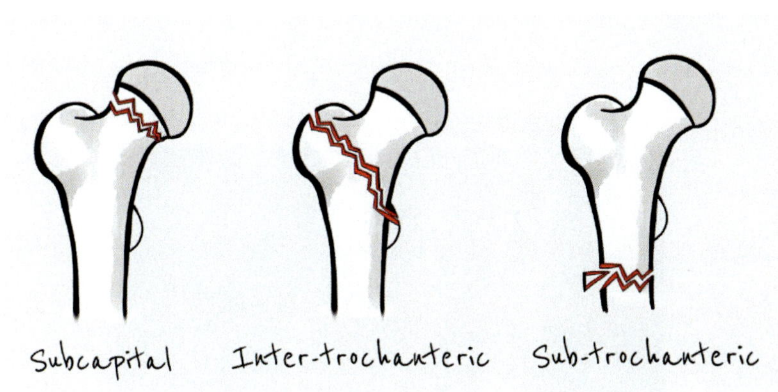

Figure 5. *Neck of femur fracture classification: 'subcapital (intracapsular)', intertrochanteric (extracapsular) and subtrochanteric (extracapsular).*

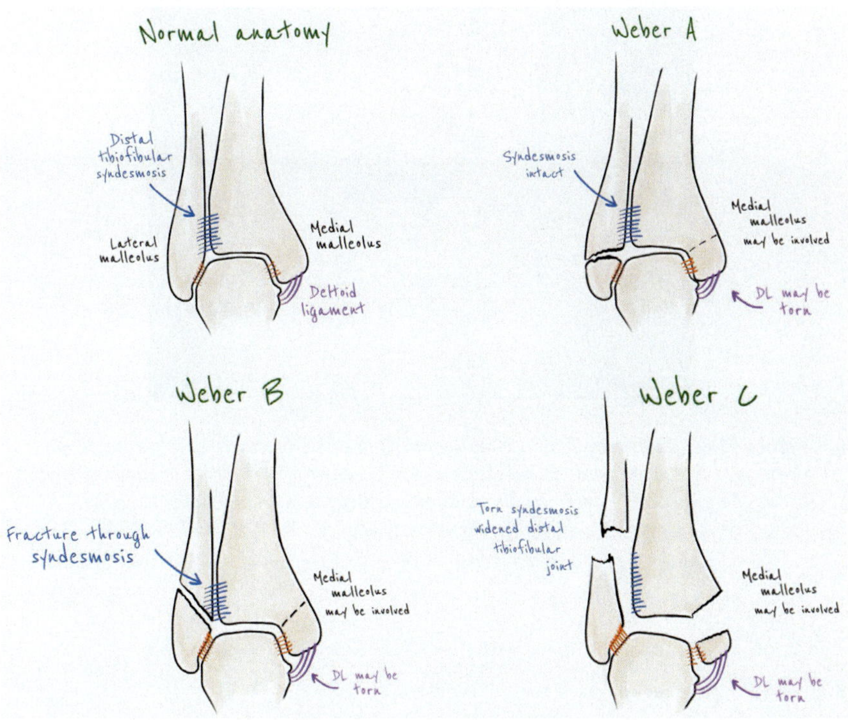

Figure 6. *Ankle fracture patterns and associated ligamentous injuries.*

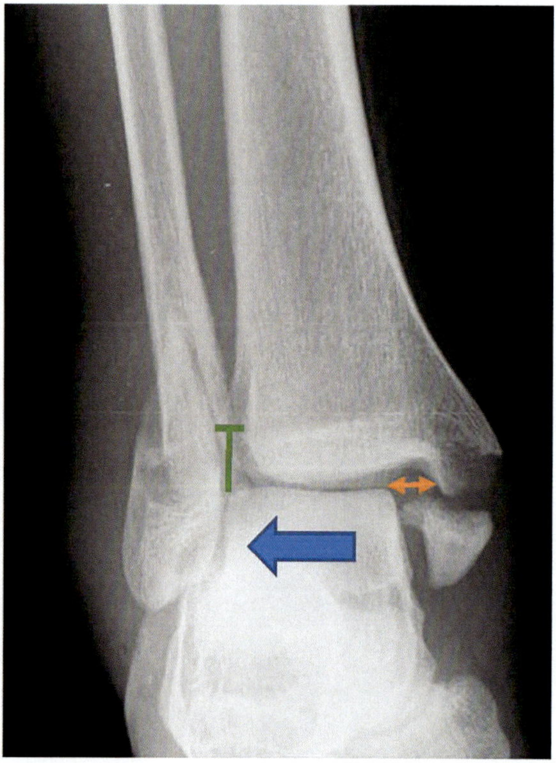

Figure 7. *AP Radiography of a bimalleolar right ankle fracture. blue arrow=Talar shift, orange = increased medial clear space, green=tib/fib overlap, measured 1cm above the joint line (<5mm is abnormal on mortice view XR) (Wikipedia, 2019).*

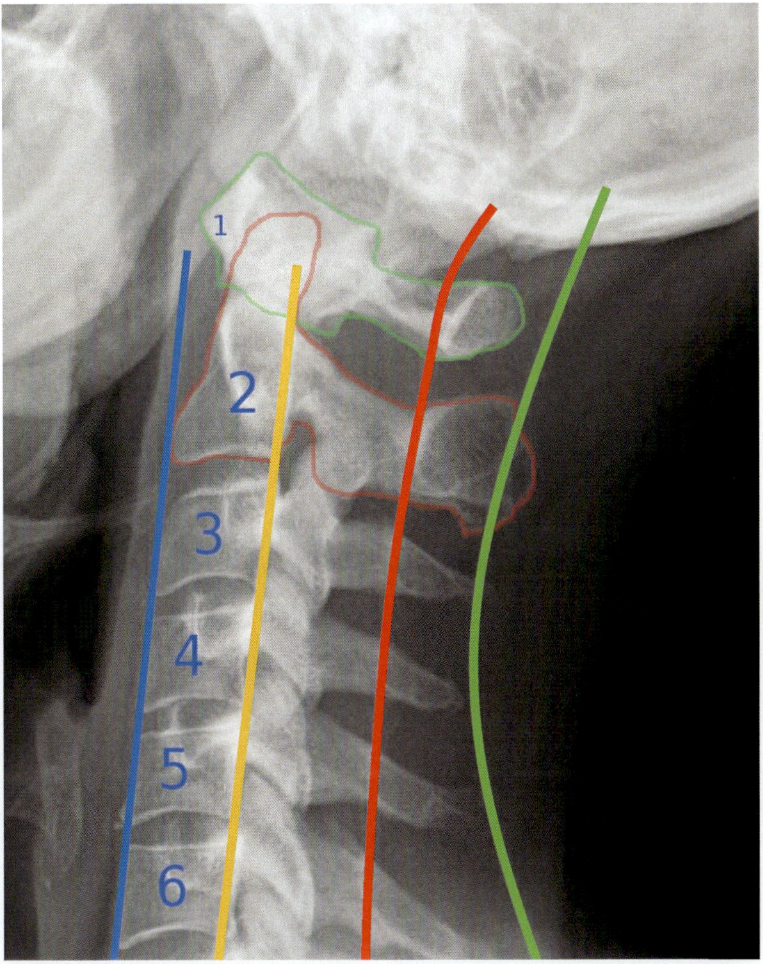

Figure 10. *Lateral XR of the Cervical spine, with each vertebrae numbered and lines to demonstrate: anterior vertebral line (blue), posterior vertebral line (yellow), spino-laminar line (red), posterior spinous line (green) (Wikipedia, 2019).*

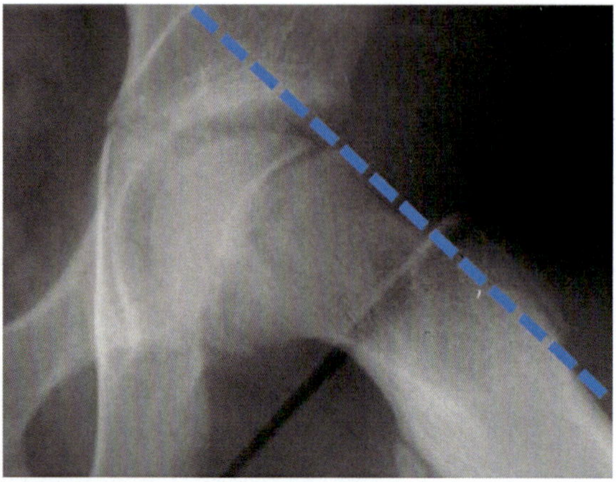

Figure 12. *Frog leg lateral radiograph of paediatric left hip. Klein's line drawn along superior aspect of femoral neck – A slipped upper femoral epiphysis is evident as the line does not intersect the femoral head. (annotated original image, (Annotated original image from, Wikipedia, 2019)*

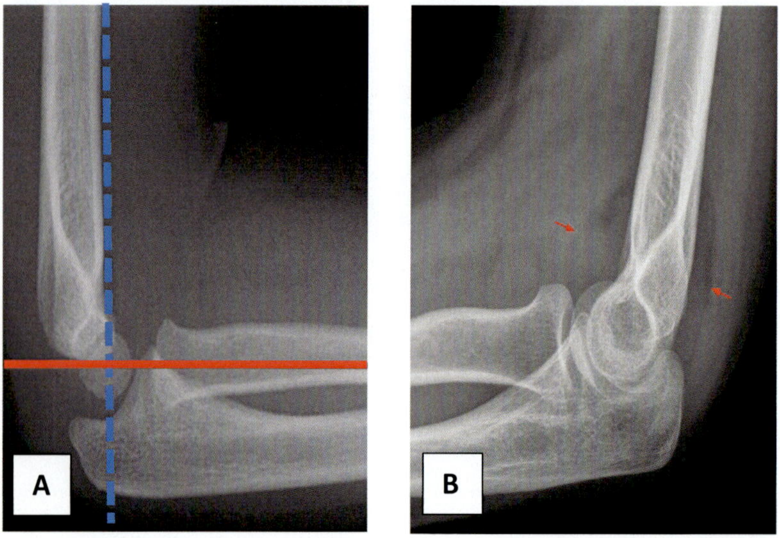

Figure 13. *a) Lateral radiograph of an uninjured skeletally immature elbow. Red = radiocapitellar line, blue = anterior humeral line b) Lateral radiography of a skeletally mature elbow, demonstrating anterior and posterior fat pad signs. (Annotated original image from, Wikipedia, 2019)*

Chapter 8: Urology

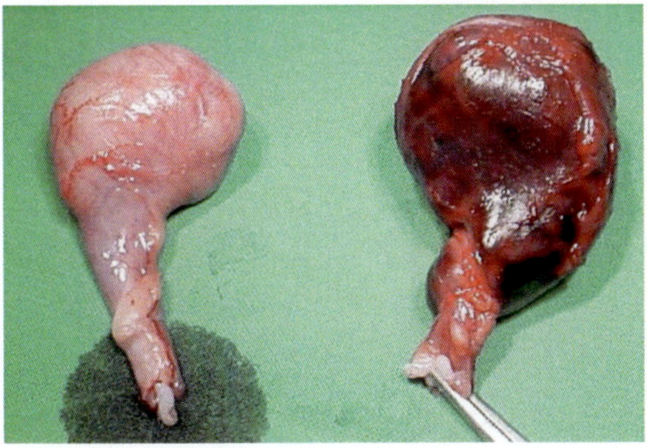

Figure 2. *An animal demonstration comparing testicular torsion. Normal, Left & Torted, Right.*

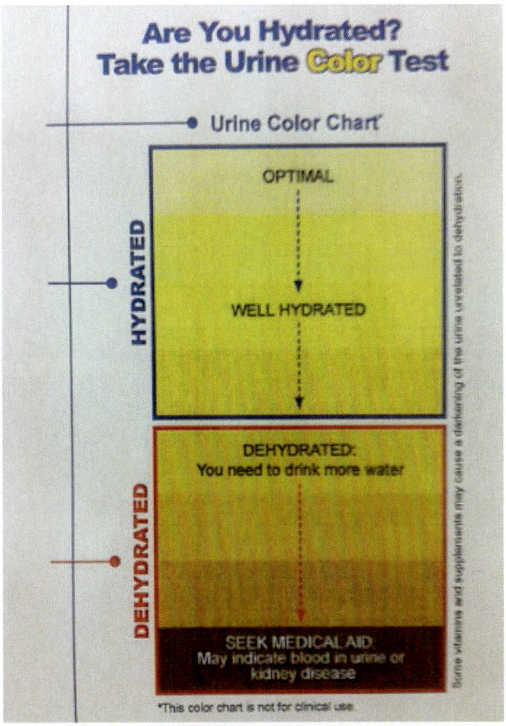

Figure 12. *Public patient information notice on urine colour.*

CHAPTER 6

PLASTIC SURGERY

MARK MIKHAIL & SALLY JAY

Abstract
Section 1 – Introduction
Section 2 – Anatomy of the upper limb
Section 4 – Infection
Paronychia
Felon
Bites
Flexor sheath infection
Necrotising Fasciitis
Section 5 – Burns
Section 6 – Amputations
Section 7 – Open Fractures
Hand open fractures
Lower limb open fractures
Section 8 – Extravasation injury
Section 9 – Flap monitoring
Section 10 – Scores and calculations in plastic surgery
Section 11 – Guidelines for referrals and management

Abstract

Plastic surgery is rarely covered in undergraduate training and often underestimated by junior doctors. On-call shifts can be stressful and busy due to the diversity of injuries and pathologies that are referred, in combination with a very high patient turnover. Although patients tend to be young and medically fit, presenting with traumatic injuries that can be managed in a day case setting, it is vital to be aware of key life and limb threatening pathologies that may also present.

This chapter covers common referrals that a Senior House Officer can expect to receive whilst on-call and will provide safe and effective methods to triage and manage patients efficiently. Common injuries covered are nail bed and pulp injuries, hand soft tissue injuries and fractures, lower limb soft tissue injuries, bite injuries and minor burns. Plastic surgery emergencies covered include resuscitation burns, compartment syndrome in the limbs, necrotising fasciitis and the failing free flap.

Finally, a key practical skill needed for plastic surgical on-calls is the ability to effectivity administer local anaesthetic to facilitate wound exploration. Herein we provide some helpful tips and tricks on how to achieve this.

Section 1: Introduction

When cross covering a different specialty, it is useful to know about the logistics of the job and in plastic surgery in particular, how to appropriately manage the many and varied referrals you will receive. This section, whilst no substitute for induction processes and formal handovers, is aimed at addressing those key areas and forms a list of questions you may find it useful to ask of the colleague from whom you are taking over.

Senior Cover

1. Who is the Consultant on call?
2. Who is the Specialist Registrar on call?
    a. Are they on site? If not, what is their distance to the hospital?
    b. What is their best contact – bleep and ideally mobile phone number

Referrals

1. What local hospitals refer to this hospital?
2. Are we a Burns Facility, Unit or Centre? (what TBSA (see later section on burns) burns do we take in adults and children?) - if not, to where do we refer? and is it ED direct referral?
3. Are we a trauma unit?
4. How are patients booked into clinics? Is this something I do, or do ED and minor injuries have direct booking access?
5. Are there any local pathways that ED should be following and that I can use?

Conditions

1. Do we accept abscesses? If so, what areas of the body?
2. Who does the initial Fournier's/ Necrotising Fasciitis debridement?
3. What fractures do we see/manage? (E.g. who takes carpal bone fractures?)
4. Who manages diabetes, or peripheral vascular disease related leg/foot wounds? (Likely to be the vascular surgeons)
5. Who manages facial injuries - lacerations, fractures, infections?
6. Who manages compartment syndrome (with/without fracture bone)?
7. Which team manages cellulitis of the upper or lower limb?

Miscellaneous

1. Are there any patients expected?
2. Are any patients going to theatre?
3. Are there any unwell patients on the ward?
4. Are there any patients who have had free flaps in the past 48hours?
5. How do I book cases for theatre?
6. How do I do a Group and save?
7. How do I access local microbiology guidelines?
8. Where does handover take place?

Section 2: Anatomy of the upper limb

Knowledge of the anatomy of the hand is fundamental to a thorough examination and assessment. A complete description or diagrammatic representation is beyond the scope of this book but here are a few key diagrams that will elicit points of note.

Simple diagrams:

Figure 1. *Hand and forearm – dermatomes (volar and dorsal)*
See colour centrefold for this image.

Figure 2. *Major forearm nerves and arteries*
See colour centrefold for this image.

Figure 3. *FDP and FDS anatomy and examination*
See colour centrefold for this image.

During a Plastic surgery on call you will be referred a large variety of patients, with the bulk of them having suffered hand trauma – there is also a huge spectrum of severity/urgency.

Many patients can be seen in an emergency clinic the following day(s) and these patients are not covered in this section. Here we focus on those patients who need to be seen and treated as a matter of urgency with the aim of providing you with the essential information to both recognise these patients and manage them appropriately.

ATLS Principles - see chapter 7.

Section 3: Infections

Paronychia

The most common hand infection. Infection of the perionychium that can also track beneath the nail-plate. Pressure necrosis can lead to death of the nailfold and nailbed. They are often incredibly painful due to the swelling and pressure effect.

Signs: Hot, red, swollen, pus collection

Management:

- Mild – oral antibiotics
- Moderate/Severe – Contact Senior as will need surgical drainage. You can perform this under a ring block if you have been trained and are competent to do so. Send a sample of the pus to the microbiology lab.

Felon

Pulp space infection

Signs: Pulp hot, swollen and exquisitely tender

Management:

- Contact Senior as will need surgical drainage.
- You can perform this under a ring block if you have been trained and are competent to do so. Send a sample of the pus to the microbiology lab.

Bites

A significant proportion of your time on call will be spent managing bites. The majority of these are from household pets (cats and dogs) but you will also be required to manage human bites as well as other exotic animals. If in doubt about an animal bite containing a toxin - Toxbase should be consulted as well as your Senior for advice.

General management:

- Wash out (No anaesthetic *vs.* Local Anaesthetic [LA] *vs.* General Anaesthetic [GA])
- Antibiotics (oral *vs.* IV)
- Tetanus vaccination
- +/- admission*

*If the wound is infected at the time of presentation admit the patient, start IV antibiotics and inform your Senior.
If there is suspicion of structural damage, discuss with your Senior.

Dog bites

90% of animal bites are domestic dog bites (Griego et al. 1995; Sacks, Kresnow, and Houston 1996). Dog bites are considered less dangerous than cat bites from an infection point of view due to a number of factors but dogs are more powerful and can cause significant damage to tissue, especially in a sustained attack, or in the case of a child (Morgan and Palmer 2007). The dog's jaw is incredibly powerful and can clamp down. This will often cause a degloving injury and devitalise tissue. The pathogens involved are similar to human bites, including mixed aerobes, anaerobes but also *Pasteurella* species (Talan et al. 1999).

Management: As above – general management

Cat Bites

Cat bites have a few properties that make them potentially more dangerous than dog bites, especially to an unsuspecting doctor. Their teeth are long, thin and sharp. They penetrate deeply but the wound will often look innocuous and may appear to be healing on review. Cat bites have a similar bacterial profile to dog bites.

Management: As above – general management

Human bites

Mixture of organisms, the majority being *Staphyloccous aureus*, *Streptococcus viridians* and mixed anaerobes.

Mechanisms:

- Deliberately bitten by assailant
- Punching someone else - ***"Fight Bite"***
    - The tooth penetrates the skin and can breach the extensor tendon and enter the metacarpal phalangeal joint (MCPJ). Mouth flora are inoculated into the wound and joint.
- Patients are often reluctant to reveal the history. The following signs should raise suspicion:
    - Wound overlying MCPJ
    - An irregular wound
    - Erythema, pus, swelling, pain, surgical emphysema – depending on timing
    - Pain on axial compression of the joint if the joint is involved and infected

Initial Management includes:

1. XR as there may be a fracture, or a foreign body such as a tooth
2. Microbiology swab if wound discharging
3. Admission
4. Elevation

5. IV antibiotics
6. Contact Senior and theatres, as needs urgent washout under GA
7. Contact tracing – test patient and if possible source (person causing bite) for Hepatitis B, C and HIV. Risk assess. Liaise with microbiology regarding vaccinations/prophylaxis

Flexor sheath infection

Early diagnosis and operative management is fundamental (Clark, 2003).

All tendons are within a sheath that allows low friction gliding of the tendon, but also spread of infection. If infection is not managed in a timely fashion, the sheath rapidly adheres to the tendon causing a permanently stiff finger. With increased pressure and pus in the sheath, there is ischaemic necrosis of the tendon and the digit itself can be threatened. Due to the anatomy of the sheath, the infection can also continue to spread rapidly, into the palm.

This is a clinical diagnosis. Your suspicions should be raised with a history of penetrating trauma to the flexor surface of the finger and when the following signs are present:

Kanavel's signs:
1. Fusiform swelling of the digit (sausage-like appearance)
2. Digit held in partial flexion
3. Tenderness along the volar aspect of the finger
4. Pain on passive extension of the digit

Management:
If you are suspicious of this diagnosis then contact your Senior immediately and begin to ready the patient for theatre by ensuring the following:

1. Patient must be kept NBM
2. Routine bloods and blood cultures if systemically unwell/pyrexial
3. Strict elevation in a Bradford sling
4. Broad spectrum antibiotics – according to local guidelines
5. Consent for theatre – if you are trained and competent to do so.
6. Adequate analgesia – this is a painful condition

Necrotising Fasciitis ('Nec Fasc')

Necrotising fasciitis is a rapidly progressive soft tissue infection that is fatal if not treated promptly and appropriately (Hasham et al. 2005; Angoules et al. 2007). It is usually polymicrobial (type 1), if monomicrobial (type 2), the most common culprit is Group A β Haemolytic Streptococci.

The treatment is invariably:

- Resuscitation
- **Urgent** debridement
- Antibiotics

History – Risk factors:

- Diabetes, immunocompromised
- Recent surgery – especially contaminated surgery e.g. bowel
- Recent trauma/microtrauma
- Multiple co-morbidities

Symptoms:

- Severe pain
- Unwell

Signs:

- Features of sepsis: tachycardia, hypotension, pyrexia, confusion.
- Skin changes: Tender, Erythema, Oedema, Induration, Blistering, Crepitus, Fixed staining

Biochemical markers:

- Infection: raised WCC and CRP
- Tissue hypoperfusion: raised lactate, renal failure

Management:
Discuss these referrals with your Senior **immediately**. If the referral is from another hospital then usually the initial, lifesaving debridement needs to occur at the referring hospital – your Senior may need liaise with the referring unit to ensure patient safety.

If you are suspicious of the diagnosis ensure the following (Inc. Sepsis 6):

1. Contact your Senior immediately.
2. Sufficient IV access – Two wide bore cannulae
3. Bloods including – Blood cultures, FBC, CRP, LFTs, U&Es, Lactate, Clotting, Group and Save, ABG: Calculate **LRINEC score** (Wong et al. 2004) (see scores and calculations section)
4. IV antibiotics – broad spectrum according to local microbiology guidelines – early advice from microbiologist
5. Oxygen
6. IV fluid resuscitation
7. Catheterisation and strict fluid balance
8. Mark erythema – to know if this has extended (very likely to between you reviewing and Senior review, such is the progression in severe cases)
9. Adequate analgesia
10. Book for theatre – contact anaesthetist
11. Alert ITU team to the likely admission post operatively
12. Consent the patient if you are trained and competent to do so. You will be explaining the need for extensive debridement beyond the obvious area. The patient must be aware of the severity of the condition, including the risk of death.
13. Your Senior may ask you to gather equipment for the "finger sweep" test

Section 4: Burns

Burns care is usually very well supported in the UK with a clear pathway depending on size and site of burn. Care is distributed into facilities, units and centres, which deal with increasingly complex burns respectively. It is crucial to know at the start of your shift, what type of burn service you are covering. Be aware that in a Burns Unit or Burns Centre, experienced nurses will provide you with invaluable support and advice.

Discussion with local Burns service should occur in the following scenarios (as advised by the London and South East England Burn Network (LSEBN 2015b)):

Cause:

- Inhalational injury
- Deep dermal and full thickness burns

- Electrical
- Chemical
- Burns with trauma

Affected area:

- Face, hands, genitals, feet, joints, scalp, ears
- Circumferential

Size – TBSA:

- >1% TBSA in children
- >3% TBSA in adults

Age:

- Neonates (<28 days old)

Wound:

- Not healed within two weeks
- Infected

Also:

- Suspected non-accidental injury (NAI)
- Progressive non-burn skin loss (TENS, SSS)
- Significant co-morbidity, or immunocompromise
- Friction burns with full thickness skin loss
- Cold burns with full thickness skin loss
- Unwell children with a burn

We advise that all cases are discussed with your Senior before accepting the referral. You will need to establish whether your service is the correct place for the management of the patient. If management would be more appropriate at a different hospital, the accident and emergency department will often make the onward referral.

Burn care starts pre-hospital and within 3 hours of the injury there is still the opportunity to provide first aid – this can impact burn depth and surface area. First aid involves putting any scald, flame or contact burn under cool running tap water for 20 minutes. For chemical burns this period of irrigation lasts until the pH has been normalised and often requires copious running water with caution not to cause hypothermia.

Information that you need to gather from the history is as follows:

1. Time of burn
2. Burning agent (temperature, voltage, pH etc)
3. Clothing worn at time and if removed
4. First aid given and for how long
5. Is there a risk of inhalational injury?
6. Tetanus immunization status
7. Past medical history

In Paediatric burns:

8. Any social worker involvement
9. Any suspicion of non-accidental injury

Minor burns

Assess the patient in the following way:

1. Give adequate analgesia to enable a more comfortable assessment and dressings
2. Check tetanus immunization status
3. Remove any clothing or jewellery, especially in hand burns
4. Clean the burn with aqueous chlorhexidine or saline – removing all loose non-viable tissue, blisters and debris
5. Assess depth of burn and TBSA (see below)
6. Dress with a non-adherent dressing according to local guidance e.g. jelonet or mepetel, followed by absorbent dressing to absorb exudate, especially in the first 72 hours.
7. Review every 3-5 days

Severe Burns: >15% TBSA in adults >10% TBSA in children and the elderly

These patients must be assessed according to ATLS/Emergency Management of Severe Burns (EMSB) principles in an ABCDE fashion, taking into consideration that the burn can be just one injury in a polytrauma setting. You should call your Senior after you get the call, not when the patient has arrived, as any delay can increase morbidity and mortality, especially in the presence of circumferential full thickness burns.

Airway:

- Suspect inhalational injury if the history suggests an enclosed space
- Carbonaceous/sooty sputum, or deposits in oropharyngeal cavity
- Deep facial or neck burns
- Change in voice
- Respiratory distress (stridor, wheeze, shortness of breath)
- Hair singe – nostrils, eyes, mouth
- Facial swelling, upper airway swelling

Breathing:

- COHb level
- Administer 100% FiO2 if any inhalational concern, whilst ongoing assessment continues
- Arterial blood gas
- Circumferential on chest - discuss with Senior immediately.

Circulation:

- Establish IV access – two large bore cannulae in unburned skin if possible
- Take baseline bloods – including cross-matching the patient. May also need CK and Drug/Toxicology screen

Disability:

- Assess pain and give adequate analgesia - this is likely to be in the form of IV opiates in the first instance.

Exposure – do this with caution not to cause hypothermia:

- Clean burn as above
- Assess burn depth and percentage surface area
- Medical photography

Fluids:

- Measure, or estimate, patient's weight
- Parkland's formula used for fluid resuscitation requirement:
    - 2-4mls x weight (in Kg) x TBSA (%)
    - Half of this given during the first 8 hours from the time of the burn
    - Remaining half in the next 16 hours
    - Adjust this according to urine output and fluid status aiming for:
        - 0.5-1ml/kg/hr Adults
        - 1ml/kg/hr Children

Assessing Depth and TBSA of burn:

Depth:

Figure 4. *Assessment of burn depth – Taken from the LSEBN Burn Depth Assessment Guidance* (LSEBN 2015a)
See colour centrefold for this image.

TBSA:

- Hand (patients): the palm of the hand is approximately 1% of the TBSA
- Rule of 9's for Adults: 9% for each arm, 18% for each leg, 9% for head,18% for front torso, 18% for back torso.
- Rule of 9's for Children: 9% for each arm, 14% for each leg, 18% for head, 18% for front torso, 18% for back torso.
- Lund and Browder Chart (See charts section below)
- Phone Application available on app store – 'Mersey Burns' (see chapter 11)

Toxic Shock Syndrome:
Toxic shock syndrome (TSS), a toxin-mediated disease, is a rare but life-threatening condition and is the most common cause of death in children with small burns.

Symptoms/Signs include:

- Temperature >38 degrees
- Rash
- General malaise
- Diarrhoea and vomiting
- Tachycardia
- Tachypnoea
- Hypotension
- Poor UO

Management:

- In conjunction with paediatricians and paediatric intensive care/ high dependency teams
- Fluid Resus + IV Antibiotics + FFP

Section 5: Amputations

The plastic surgery team will be involved in the revascularisation/replantation of partially or fully amputated digits and limbs.

There are a number of key questions to ask and assessments to make when evaluating these patients that you will want to relay to the Senior, to assist in making important decisions. Whenever you take a referral, or see a patient, the following information needs to be ascertained:

1. Referring hospital
2. Age of patient
3. Time since injury
4. Amputated part
5. Level of the injury? E.g. "through the middle of the middle phalanx of the index finger"
6. Mechanism - Clean cut? crush?
7. Where is the part? What condition is it in?
8. Co-morbidities and previous medical history
9. Smoking - estimate of quantity
10. Profession of patient and relevant hobbies
11. Handedness
12. When did they last eat or drink?
13. Does the patient have any other injuries? Is there a plan for surgical intervention for them?

Generally, discuss these referrals immediately, and usually before accepting, with your Senior on call. When you accept the patient, ask the referring department to do the following:

1. Place the amputated tissue in a damp (with saline) gauze, inside a bag, that is placed in a container with iced water.
2. Keep the patient NBM
3. Have the patient 'blue-lighted' over.
4. If it will not significantly delay, ask the referring department to perform XRs of the part and limb and give one dose of IV antibiotics.

Ensure you manage patient expectation, in particular in relation to digits. Sometimes ED will tell the patient they are being referred to plastics for the part to be reattached – sometimes it is not technically possible and sometimes it is not advisable. It is helpful if the patient knows this from the start.

Time is of the essence when a body part has been amputated. Due to the lack of muscle in the digits there is a relatively low metabolic demand and so 'ischaemic time' can be longer and replant still be successful; although, the sooner the patient can get to theatre the better. For hands/limbs with muscular components, generally 6 hours from time of injury is the rule.

The surgery is long and requires significant skill. Patients post operatively should be managed in the same way as a free flap (see below), with regular reviews and documentation of status of the replanted part.

Section 6: Open fractures

An open fracture is a break in a bone which is associated with a wound/soft tissue defect. They are often secondary to high energy trauma and are typically caused by road traffic collisions. If in doubt, a soft tissue wound in close proximity to an open fracture should be treated as such until proven otherwise.

Hand open fractures

As an SHO covering plastic surgery the majority of open fractures you will come across will be of the hand. Key steps in the emergency department carried out by the on call SHO can prevent significant complications.

* Please note this does not apply to nailbed injuries which is a laceration of the nailbed with an underlying distal phalanx fracture – these can almost always be managed on an outpatient basis *

1. Ensure adequate imaging – AP, oblique and true lateral X-Ray
2. Assess the soft tissue and degree of damage
3. Assess the function, perfusion and sensation of the hand for other damaged structures
4. Take note of the degree of contamination (farm/factory injury etc)
5. Check Tetanus vaccination status and vaccinate appropriately
6. Contact your Senior
7. Admit the patient
8. Begin intravenous antibiotics – check local guidelines
9. Give adequate analgesia
10. If not for formal washout that day/night and competent to do so infiltrate local anaesthetic and irrigate the wound thoroughly with normal saline or a running tap.
11. Manipulate the fracture if competent, having discussed with your Senior (under local anaesthetic)
12. Place in a Volar slab plaster of Paris
13. Keep elevated in a Bradford sling
14. Book for theatre for a formal debridement, washout +/- fracture fixation +/- Soft tissue reconstruction

Lower limb open fracture (and upper limb except hand)

Open fractures of the lower limb should be managed in a trauma centre with joint involvement from orthopaedic and plastic surgical teams (see chapter 7). The principles are outlined below and extracted from the British Orthopaedic Association Standards for Trauma (BOAST) 4 guidelines (Nanchahal et al. 2009). Initial ATLS assessment and resuscitation should be done in the first instance, followed by a more focussed examination and management.

1. Early (ideally within 1 hour of injury) prophylactic antibiotics should be given and the antibiotic of choice is co-amoxiclav (1.2g 8 hourly), or a cephalosporin (e.g. Cefuroxime 1.5g)
2. Examine limb, including documentation of vascular and neurological status. This should be repeated systematically
3. Re-align limb and splint

4. Remove gross contaminants - no informal washout at bedside should be carried out.
5. Medical photography
6. Dress with saline-soaked gauze and cover with occlusive film

Key points to document
1. Colour
2. Capillary refill time
3. Compartments - soft/tense, pain on passive stretch
4. Sensation
5. Movement
6. Pulses
7. Temperature

Patient will need combined orthoplastic surgery - time frame determined by severity of injury. Work the patient up for theatre.

Section 7: Extravasation

Extravasation is the accidental leakage of IV fluids from an IV drip in the vein into the surrounding tissue. It is often noticed due to pain during the time of intravenous administration, however, can present late. The injuries are on a large spectrum and although very few will need any intervention, all should be treated seriously and assessed rapidly.

The management will depend on several key things:

- *Fluid involved* – It is important to determine which category the fluid falls into:
    - *Vesicant:* drugs which are capable of causing pain, inflammation and blistering of the local skin and underlying structures: if left untreated may lead to tissue necrosis
    - Irritant: drugs which are capable of causing inflammation, irritation or pain at the site of extravasation but rarely cause tissue necrosis
    - Non-vesicant: inert or neutral compounds that do not cause inflammation or damage but can cause pain.
- *Volume involved*
- *Time from extravasation*

Key points when taking a referral:

1. Solution administered and concentration
2. Volume administered
3. Timing of extravasation
4. Location of venous access
5. Current state of skin – symptoms and signs (coolness, swelling, tenderness, poor cap refill, numbness, erythema)

Advice to referring team:

1. Leave cannula in and aspirate
2. Elevate limb
3. Compress (warm/cold – there is no strong evidence between the two, however, different hospitals will have different guidelines).

Management:

1. Assess patient promptly
2. Assessment will determine whether the area needs flushing (best done within 2 hours of extravasation). Flushing involves infiltration with LA and hyaluronidase, followed by 4-8 punctures and normal saline flush (this is known as the Gault technique). Proceed if you have been trained and are competent to do this and are confident with your assessment, otherwise, contact your Senior.

Section 8: Useful Techniques in the emergency setting

Pressure dressing to stop bleeding

Pressure dressing is a simple skill that is often done poorly and can generate late night calls from the emergency department to stop a patient's wound from bleeding.

If you are in a situation where the bleeding is significant, it is often more valuable to gain control of this whilst you simultaneously assess the complete picture in an ABCDE fashion. Often stemming the bleeding will halt the panic as well as prevent hypotension and a drop in Hb.

The equation that underlies the principle is:

$$Pressure = \frac{Force}{Area}$$

This means that more pressure can be generated if the force is placed through a smaller area. This is a common mistake in the inexperienced when several tight bandages have been placed around the entire limb or scalp uniformly.

Practical steps:

1. Ask for help from your nursing colleagues – this can be a two-person job.
2. Make sure the patient has been given analgesia.
3. Identify the bleeding point or area.
4. Place your sterile gloved finger over the suspected area and assess whether this has stemmed the bleeding.
5. If it has, then move on, if not return to step 2
6. Take a piece of gauze and fold it into a small square
7. Place this over the bleeding point
8. Place another piece of gauze, slightly larger than the first over this
9. Over this second piece, place a further piece of gauze unfolded
10. Hold with a bandage

The very important caveat to this is when there is suspicion of a significant arterial bleed from a major vessel, for example the brachial artery: contact your Senior immediately.

Local anaesthetic ring and field

You will often need to give local anaesthetic to aid examination, provide analgesia, perform washouts or carry out simple procedures.

There are multiple different local anaesthetics. All of them work on the sodium channels and all work intracellularly.

Common local anaesthetic choices:

- Short acting e.g. Lignocaine OR Long acting e.g. bupivacaine
- ‘Plain’ or containing adrenaline (often in a 1:200,000 ratio).

A common choice is a mixture of short and long acting – usually with adrenaline (the adrenaline allows a bigger dose/volume to be used and vasoconstriction which retains the LA at the site for longer and can also facilitate surgery by limiting the amount of blood in the surgical field.

Local anaesthetics can be painful to inject, depending on site. You can add 8.4% sodium bicarbonate to improve the pain. This is only done with lignocaine/lidocaine and is in a 10:1 ratio (local:bicarbonate)

Dosing:
Local anaesthetics can cause toxicity if too much is given and so knowing the correct dosing is key:

- Ligocaine 'plain' - 3mg/kg max dose
- Ligocaine with adrenaline - 7mg/kg max dose
- Bupivicaine ('plain' or with adrenaline) – 2mg/kg max dose

Ring block:
This is a really useful skill to learn – ask your Senior to train you in this skill and only perform it when you are competent to do so. There are several ways to carry out a ring block and the key is to use a method that works for you consistently. One example is shown in the diagram below:

Figure 5. *Ring block and field block local anaesthetic techniques*
See colour centrefold for this image.

Field Block:
This is a useful skill to master in enabling you to wash out wounds in a pain-free manner.

Section 9: Free flaps

Most elective patients will need minimal input out of hours, unless there is a concern. However, free flaps need more intensive monitoring.

Free flaps involve the transfer of tissue with its blood supply to a distant location and joining the blood supply to a recipient blood supply. The tissue itself can be composed of skin and fat, muscle, nerve, bone – or a combination thereof. Common examples of free flaps are:

- Orthoplastic: to cover a soft tissue defect in an open lower limb fracture
- Breast reconstruction: abdominal based flap (MS-TRAM/DIEP)
- Head and Neck reconstruction, post cancer resection

Flap Monitoring

It is important to establish at the start of your shift if any patients have had free flaps in the past 48 hours. If they have, it is sensible to review the patients and the flaps early, ideally with your Senior initially, in order that you are better able to assess any changes during the course of your shift. Read the op note - instructions will often be quite clearly documented e.g. permissible parameters for BP or Hb, thromboprophylaxis plan and blood tests.

The patients have gone through significant operations. Even in the fastest hands the anaesthetic time is many hours. It is important to monitor the following:

General factors

1. Urine output and fluid status – tailor fluids accordingly
2. Analgesia – patients will often have a PCA
3. Bloods results – there may be a request for a post op Hb and HCT with target parameters

Flap factors – this depends on whether the flap is a muscle flap or a fasciocutaneous flap i.e. has skin to see.

	Muscle	Fasciocutaneous
Colour	Healthy muscle with red/orange tinge	'Normal' (for that patient) skin colour
Cap refill	Not applicable	2 seconds Rapid can represent venous problem Prolonged can represent arterial problem
Temperature	Warm	Warm
Doppler signal*	Present	Present

Table 1. *Flap observations*

A change in the flap status is also very important

There are different types of Doppler

- External – listen on the surface of the skin or muscle
- Internal – a tiny probe is adjacent to the venous anastomosis

Remember the nursing staff usually have specialist skills in managing free flaps and provide a wealth of information

If there are any issues, or you are unsure, rapidly escalate to your Senior. If they are not available, escalate up the ranks to the **operating surgeon,** as more often than not they would want to be informed about any concerns.

If the flap is struggling, then there is a need to act quickly to try to salvage it - prepare the patient for theatre in the normal way and contact the anaesthetist on call.

Section 10: SCORES and calculations for plastic surgery

This is a non-exhaustive list of commonly used assessment and management tools. All of these have their drawbacks and should always be used with caution.

Gustilo Anderson – Modified classification of open fractures (Gustilo and Anderson 1976; Gustilo, Merkow, and Templeman 1990).

Gustillo Type	**I**	**II**	**IIIA**	**IIIB**	**IIIC**
Wound Size	≤1cm	1-10cm	Usually >10cm	Usually >10cm	Usually >10cm
Soft Tissue Damage	Minimal	Moderate	Extensive	Extensive	Extensive
Contamination	Clean	Moderate	Extensive	Extensive	Extensive
Fracture Pattern	Simple pattern with minimal comminution	Moderate comminution	Severe comminution or segmental fractures	Severe comminution or segmental fractures	Severe comminution or segmental fractures
Periosteal stripping	No	No	Yes	Yes	Yes

Skin coverage	Local coverage	Local coverage	Local Coverage	Free tissue flap or rotational flap coverage	Typically free flap
Neurovascular injury	No	No	No	No	Arterial damage requiring repair

Table 2. *Gustillo-Anderson Classifiction of open tib/fib fractures*

Lund and Browder chart – this is the most accurate way to assess burn TBSA as it takes the patient's age into consideration. *Adapted from Grabb and Smith: Plastic Surgery* (Klein 2007)

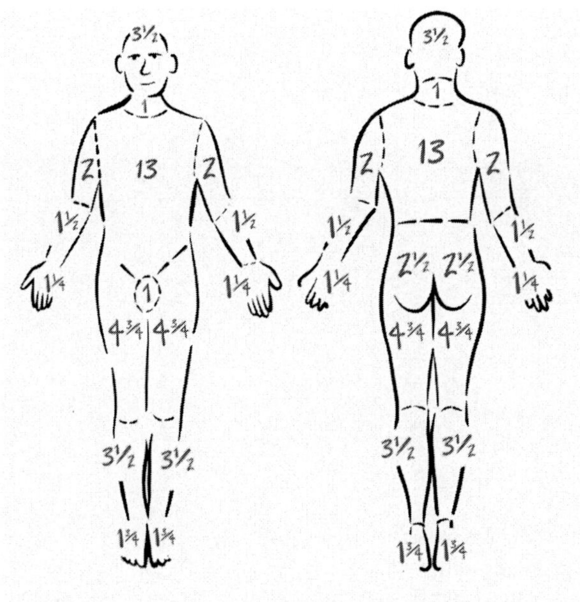

Figure 6. *Lund and Browder diagram for adults – The percentage values for the head, upper and lower legs are then adjusted for depending on the age of the child.* (*Adapted from Grabb and Smith: Plastic Surgery* [Klein 2007*])*

LRINEC – Laboratory Risk Indicator for Necrotising Fasciitis (Wong et al. 2004)

This scoring system is a tool often quoted in helping diagnose necrotising fasciitis. It can be used as an adjunct, but should not replace clinical judgment and a Senior review. It has been shown to be of limited clinical significance with high false positive and false negative rates (Neeki et al. 2017; Burner et al. 2016). Notably lactate does not comprise part of this but will always be part of discussions with your Senior.

Laboratory Test, Units		Score (max 13)
C-Reactive Protein, mg/L	<150	0
	>150	4
Total white cell count, per mm^3	<15	0
	15-25	1
	>25	2
Haemoglobin, g/dL	>13.5	0
	11-13.5	1
	<11	2
Sodium, mmol/L	≥135	0
	<135	2
Creatinine, μmol/L	≤141	0
	>141	2
Glucose, mmol/L	≤10	0
	>10	1

Table 3. *LRINEC scoring*

A score of ≥6 should raise suspicion and a score of ≥ 8 *is strongly predictive of the disease*

PARKLANDS formula – For calculation of first 24 hours fluids for resuscitating large burns (Baxter 1974)

Give ½ of total in first 8 hours **(TIME STARTS is from INJURY)** 2nd ½ in next 16 hours

This should be adjusted according to parameters of fluid status, most importantly urine output and blood pressure.

Fluid Requirement = TBSA % x Weight (kg) x 2-4mL

Section 11: Guidelines for referrals and management

The Oxford University Hospitals Plastics Surgery Department have created treatment decision pathways to assist the on-call Senior House Officer triage, prioritise and manage plastics surgery emergency referrals. They can also be accessed via the free and easy to use mobile application available on the App store for iOS and Android.

Although there are some specific elements to the Oxford team (numbers to ring), this provides a helpful decision aid for the on-call doctor. Use these to discuss cases with referrers over the phone, or before you attend the patient, to give an idea of the correct and safest pathway. They will also provide a reminder for the actions that ED /referring units are required to take.

Figure 7. HIPE app interface with example of pathway for hand laceration injuries (left to right). Selected options highlighted in red.
See colour centrefold for this image.

References

Angoules, A G, G Kontakis, E Drakoulakis, G Vrentzos, M S Granick, and P V Giannoudis. 2007. "Necrotising Fasciitis of Upper and Lower Limb: A Systematic Review." *Injury* 38 (5, Supplement): S18–25. https://doi.org/https://doi.org/10.1016/j.injury.2007.10.030.

Baxter, C R. 1974. "Fluid Volume and Electrolyte Changes of the Early Postburn Period." *Clinics in Plastic Surgery* 1 (4): 693–703.

Burner, Elizabeth, Sean O Henderson, Guenevere Burke, Jeffrey Nakashioya, and Jerome R Hoffman. 2016. "Inadequate Sensitivity of Laboratory Risk Indicator to Rule Out Necrotizing Fasciitis in the Emergency Department." *The Western Journal of Emergency Medicine* 17 (3): 333–36. https://doi.org/10.5811/westjem.2016.2.29069.

Clark, Dwayne C. 2003. "Common Acute Hand Infections." *American Family Physician* 68 (11): 2167—2176. http://europepmc.org/abstract/MED/14677662.

Griego, Robert D, Ted Rosen, Ida F Orengo, and John E Wolf. 1995. "Dog,

Cat, and Human Bites: A Review." *Journal of the American Academy of Dermatology* 33 (6): 1019–29. https://doi.org/https://doi.org/10.1016/0190-9622(95)90296-1.

Gustilo, R B, and J T Anderson. 1976. "Prevention of Infection in the Treatment of One Thousand and Twenty-Five Open Fractures of Long Bones: Retrospective and Prospective Analyses." *The Journal of Bone and Joint Surgery. American Volume* 58 (4): 453–58.

Gustilo, R B, R L Merkow, and D Templeman. 1990. "The Management of Open Fractures." *The Journal of Bone and Joint Surgery. American Volume* 72 (2): 299–304.

Hasham, Saiidy, Paolo Matteucci, Paul R W Stanley, and Nick B Hart. 2005. "Necrotising Fasciitis." *BMJ* 330 (7495): 830–33. https://doi.org/10.1136/bmj.330.7495.830.

Klein, Matthew. 2007. "Thermal, Chemical, and Electrical Injuries." In *Grabb and Smith: Plastic Surgery*, edited by Robert Beasley, Sherrell Aston, Scott Bartlett, Geoffrey Gurtner, Scott Spear, and Charles Thorne, 6th ed., 135. Lippincott Williams and Wilkins (530 Walnut Street,P O Box 327, Philadelphia PA 19106-3621, United States).

LSEBN. 2015a. "Burn Depth Assessment." 2015.

—. 2015b. "Burn Referral Guidelines: Criteria for Referral." 2015. http://www.lsebn.nhs.uk/website/X13911/files/LSEBN Burns Referral Criteria.pdf.

Morgan, Marina, and John Palmer. 2007. "Dog Bites." *BMJ* 334 (7590): 413–17. https://doi.org/10.1136/bmj.39105.659919.BE.

Nanchahal, Jagdeep, Selvadurai Nayagam, Umraz Khan, Christopher Moran, Stephen Barrett, Frances Sanderson, and Ian Pallister. 2009. *Standards for the Management of Open Fractures of the Lower Limb*. Royal Society of Medicine Press.

Neeki, Michael M, Fanglong Dong, Christine Au, Jake Toy, Nima Khoshab, Carol Lee, Eugene Kwong, et al. 2017. "Evaluating the Laboratory Risk Indicator to Differentiate Cellulitis from Necrotizing Fasciitis in the Emergency Department." *The Western Journal of Emergency Medicine* 18 (4): 684–89. https://doi.org/10.5811/westjem.2017.3.33607.

Sacks, J J, M Kresnow, and B Houston. 1996. "Dog Bites: How Big a Problem?" *Injury Prevention* 2 (1): 52 LP-54. https://doi.org/10.1136/ip.2.1.52.

Talan, David A, Diane M Citron, Fredrick M Abrahamian, Gregory J Moran, and Ellie J C Goldstein. 1999. "Bacteriologic Analysis of Infected Dog and Cat Bites." *New England Journal of Medicine* 340 (2): 85–92. https://doi.org/10.1056/NEJM199901143400202.

Wong, Chin-Ho, Lay-Wai Khin, Kien-Seng Heng, Kok-Chai Tan, and

Cheng-Ooi Low. 2004. "The LRINEC (Laboratory Risk Indicator for Necrotizing Fasciitis) Score: A Tool for Distinguishing Necrotizing Fasciitis from Other Soft Tissue Infections." *Critical Care Medicine* 32 (7): 1535–41.

CHAPTER 7

TRAUMA AND ORTHOPAEDICS

OLIVER BEAUMONT & OLIVER GOSLING

Abstract
Section 1 – Principals of radiology interpretation
Section 2 – Trauma Calls
Section 3 – Principles for emergency management of fractures and dislocated joints
Section 4 – Open fractures
Section 5 – Upper limb
Distal radial fractures
Scaphoid fractures
Forearm fractures
Clavicle fractures
Scapula fractures
Floating elbow
Humeral fractures
Upper limb dislocations
Section 6 – Lower limb fractures
Neck of femur fractures
Ankle fractures
Lisfranc injuries
Tibia/ fibular fractures
Lower limb dislocations
Section 7 – Pelvic fractures
Section 8 – Septic joints
Section 9 – Osteomyelitis
Section 10 – Compartment syndrome
Section 11 – Spinal Injuries
C-spine
Thoracic spine
Section 12 – Paediatric orthopaedics
Septic hip
Disorders of the hip
Paediatric trauma

Abstract

Trauma and orthopaedics (T&O) can be a surprisingly difficult specialty to cross-cover due to the complexity of both the patients and injuries presenting to on-call teams. The patient populations are often either frail with multiple medical co-morbidities or young who have sustained high energy injuries.

This chapter summarises the key principles for approaching and assessing trauma patients using the advance trauma life support principles. Often the on-call trauma and orthopaedic senior house officer is expected to take an active role in trauma calls, including conducting primary or secondary surveys. This can be daunting but is achievable with a systematic, methodical approach. The chapter then covers common referrals including open and closed fractures, joint dislocations, septic joints and major joint soft tissue injuries. Although many orthopaedic injuries can be splinted and managed in an outpatient setting it is vital to be aware of those that require admission and urgent/early intervention. This chapter will also cover the key principles in addressing paediatric orthopaedics.

Often the orthopaedic SHO is asked to give opinions on radiographs, although this can sometimes be inappropriate and may be discussed with a radiologist, it is important to have a method for approaching images in order to identify key injuries and manage them correctly. Furthermore, although more commonly performed by A&E teams, it is important for junior doctors cross covering T&O to understand the principles of fracture reductions and splinting. This chapter will cover the basic principles and provide some general tips and tricks that can be used.

Section 1: Principles of radiology interpretation

Have a system for looking at radiographs. You are likely to be asked to present them in trauma meetings and it will facilitate a succinct handover to senior colleagues. Start with name/date/age - mention if skeletally immature. Then "the obvious injury is…" State whether it is intra/extra-articular, comminuted (multi-fragmentary)/two-part, transverse/oblique/spiral. If displaced say in what way: translated, rotated, shortened/distracted or angulated.

When admitting patients with bone or joint presenting complaints radiographs are required. At least two views (Anterior-Posterior [AP] and

Lateral) should be requested. Images should be checked to ensure that they are adequate. Failure to do this may delay surgical planning. You should also always consider imaging the joint above or below and get full-length views of long bones, particularly with a history of malignancy.

Section 2: Trauma calls

Many SHOs covering Trauma and Orthopaedics will be expected to attend trauma calls. Within the modern major trauma system the more severely injured patients will go directly to tertiary centres. However, in certain scenarios, such as an unstable patient that is too far from the nearest Major Trauma Centre (MTC), multiply injured patients may arrive at any accident and emergency department and you should be prepared for a trauma call wherever you work.

Staff should be identified and clearly given roles. As the Orthopaedic SHO, your role may vary. You may be required to scribe – contemporaneously documenting who is present, patient vital signs, examination findings and interventions performed. There is often a structured booklet for this and it is worth familiarising yourself with it before your first trauma call.

You may also be asked to perform the primary survey. The safest and most universally performed method of assessing the acute trauma patient is by the Adult Trauma Life Support (ATLS) principles:

- **A – Airway**: Speak to the patient – if they speak back to you it is a good indication their airway is clear – if not, why not – is there something blocking the airway that could be removed – do they need their airway securing? This would be the time to involve the anaesthetist or alternative senior clinician with airway skills.
    - C-spine – should be considered along with airway. If the mechanism suggests there may be a c-spine injury, or the patient is complaining of neck pain, they should be 'triple immobilised' to restrict cervical spine movement in a hard C-spine collar, blocks and tape. This has often already been applied in the pre-hospital setting. It is worth getting to know the collars in your ED before you need to fit them to a patient for the first time. If the C-spine is secure, you can move on with the assessment. A diagnosis of C-spine injury does not need to be made before moving to B.

- **B – Breathing**: by this point other members of the team should have attached monitoring. The patient should be fully exposed for an adequate examination – this usually means cutting all clothes off. Check the respiratory rate and O2 sats. Check for a central trachea, signs of respiratory distress, is the chest expanding equally bilaterally – look for pneumothorax/haemothorax/tension pneumothorax. Look for obvious bruising, feel for subcutaneous crepitus, are the ribs tender? Is there a flail segment? Percuss the chest and auscultate the lungs. Don't forget to look at the posterior lateral aspects of the chest wall that are often missed.

- **C – Circulation**: Is there any obvious bleeding – think 'on the floor and 4 more' – chest, abdomen, pelvis, thigh. Check the BP and heart rate, central and peripheral capillary refill times. Feel the radial pulse – rhythm and character. Feel the carotid pulse and listen to the heart – remember Beck's triad of cardiac tamponade - muffled heart sounds, distended neck veins and hypotension with narrow pulse pressure. Inspect (for wounds, abrasions, seat belt bruises) and palpate the abdomen for tenderness to identify significant abdominal injury. Look for evidence of pelvic/femoral injury – shortened/rotated leg, perineal bruising, blood at the urethral meatus.

- **D – Disability**: Perform a swift neurological examination. What is the GCS/AVPU score? Examine the pupils. Is the patient moving all 4 limbs? Briefly assess power and sensation in all limbs. Check the Glucose.

- **E – Exposure**: Ensuring enough people are on hand, log roll the patient. Look for obvious injuries on the posterior thorax and back - palpate the spine and perform a digital rectal examination, documenting your findings - this is also a good time to remove any glass/debris from under the patient and remove the spinal board if present. Warm the patient with blanket or Bair Hugger - Remember the lethal triad – hypothermia, acidosis, coagulopathy (Figure 1).

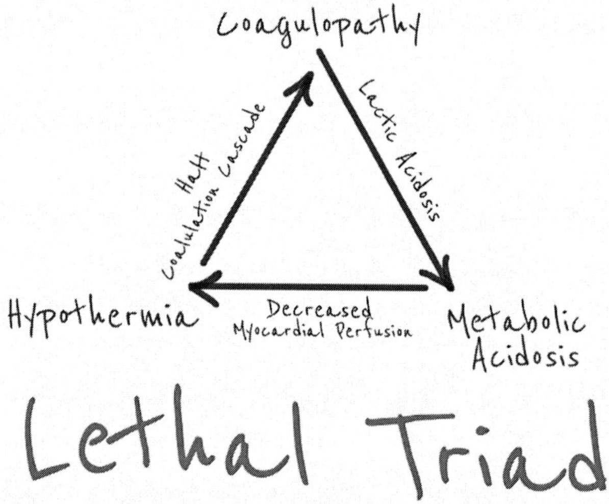

Figure 1. *The Lethal Triad observed in trauma scenarios*

If the status of the patient changes during the primary survey, re-start from the top. Remember to vocalise your findings clearly to the scribe as you go, to re-affirm to yourself and to keep the rest of the team fully informed. Your job here is to rapidly and effectively identify problems and raise them to the team. If you are not sure, ask for help.

If possible, you should try to attend the full ATLS course prior to your post as a trauma and orthopaedic SHO, however this may not be possible. If you have not attended a course, it is prudent to inform your senior team that you are not ATLS trained, so that they have an awareness of how comfortable you are in managing these situations.

Section 3: Principles for emergency management of fractures and dislocated joints

Fractures

The management of any fracture can usually be broken down into a series of generalizable steps:

1. Resuscitate the patient – as per ATLS/ABC approach.
2. Reduce the fracture
3. Hold the reduction
4. Rehabilitate

When reducing fractures in ED, ensure the patient has analgesia and is suitably sedated. You do not want to cause a patient unnecessary pain. Pain may also increase resting muscle tone which will impede adequate reduction. For some, e.g. wrist fractures, this may be nitrous oxide gas, for others deeper sedation may need senior staff with airways skills in a resus bay. If a fracture can't be adequately reduced it may need to go to theatre for formal manipulation under anaesthesia.

Reduction of certain fractures may require inline traction for several minutes – the viscoelastic properties of the soft tissue mean that they will stretch slowly over time. Have an assistant performing counter traction and remember to take your time. Think about muscles crossing joints and position the limb to reduce their effect, eg flex the knee to remove the plantarflexion force of the Achilles when attempting to reduce an ankle. Adequate initial traction will make things much easier but time goes slowly when you are standing there pulling! Usually the deforming force must first be exaggerated to 'unlock' the fracture, then, whilst maintaining traction, the distal side brought back to its correct location, using the cortex as a leverage point. You may be able to feel the fracture reducing with your thumb. Once you feel the fracture is reduced, apply a back-slab cast, then mould with three-point fixation to ensure close pressure in the correct areas (Figure 2). Pre and post-reduction you should check the neurovascular status of the limb and a check radiograph in cast is mandatory to assess the quality of the reduction.

Figure 2. *Locations for 3-point fixation in a wrist fracture. Note how the intact periosteal hinge acts to align the fracture.*
See colour centrefold for this image.

Joint dislocations

Patients will often present in pain with a deformed joint. Radiographs are required in all cases to rule out a fracture and identify the nature of the dislocation (if suspected). In all cases it is important to assess the distal neurovascular status before and after relocation.

Relocation of joints is similar to fracture reductions. Analgesia with or without sedation is key, as is an assistant. If you have not performed a relocation of that joint before then ensure you have senior supervision.

Section 4: Open fractures

Open fractures should be treated according to current British Orthopaedic Association Standards for Trauma (BOAST 4, 2017) guidelines, key points for initial management include:

- ATLS resuscitation
- Assess the limb – soft tissues, neurovascular status
- IV antibiotics and Tetanus
- Trauma CT and angiogram where indicated
- Treat arterial injuries
- Analgesia
- Photographs to document the injury (use departmental camera NOT your phone)
- Wound management – simple dressing, not for aggressive washout or debridement in the emergency department
- Splint the fracture

All open fractures should go directly to a major trauma centre (excluding digit/hand/wrist/forefoot) for further management. They may be classified according to the Gustilo and Anderson classification (see table 2 in chapter 6).

Section 5: Upper limb

Distal radial fractures

Wrist fractures are common in the elderly, but in the acute setting can often be managed by ED and brought to a fracture clinic. As with all fractures, document intact distal neurovascular status before sending the patient home.

Some fractures will require surgery, others can be managed definitively in cast. Initially a back-slab is used to allow for swelling. See back to figure 2 for a suitably moulded cast. As a rough guide, the table and associated figure below shows what bony displacement is acceptable to manage conservatively (Table 1). These should still be followed up in a fracture clinic.

Important Radiographic features in Distal Radius Fractures		
	Normal	What to accept
Radial shortening	13mm	<5mm short
Radial Inclination	23 degrees	<5 degrees change
Volar tilt	11 degrees	<5 degrees **dorsal** angulation

Table 1. *Details the normal parameters for anatomy of the distal radius and what change to accept in a displaced fracture.*

If the deformity is greater, consider further manipulation in ED. As with all fractures around joints, carefully review the radiographs for intra-articular involvement as this is often an indication for surgery. Any wrist fracture which is open or with neurovascular compromise requires admission and early discussion with a senior. Most other wrist fractures with acceptable alignment can be managed via fracture clinic. If you are unsure, discuss with a senior or keep the patients details to discuss in the morning. It is also important to assess Gilulas arcs to check carpal alignment (Figure 3). If these are abnormal consult a senior urgently.

Figure 3. *Gilulas ARCS in blue on an AP radiograph of the wrist. The red arrow points to a scaphoid waist fracture. 1 (Wikipedia, 2019)*
See colour centrefold for this image.

Scaphoid Fractures

These should really be managed by ED and sent to fracture clinic but if clinically suspicious and normal radiographs treat as a fracture and immobilise. See figure 3 above for an example of a scaphoid waist fracture.

Forearm fractures

With forearm fractures it is important to examine both the wrist and the elbow so as not to miss another fracture or dislocation. Think of the forearm like a polo mint – it normally fails in 2 places except for nightstick fractures (direct blow to the ulna). This analogy can also be applied to the pelvis and jaw.

- Monteggia – fracture proximal 1/3 ulna with dislocated head of the radius
- Galeazzi – fracture of distal 1/3 radius with dislocated distal radio-ulnar joint (DRUJ)

- Essex-Lopresti – fracture through radial head and dislocation of DRUJ with disruption of interosseous membrane.

Clavicle Fractures

Manage conservatively in the first instance and send to fracture clinic unless concern of overlying skin.

Scapula fracture

These are usually very high energy mechanism and therefore it is important to consider other injuries

Floating shoulder

If there is a fracture of the long bones either side of a joint then it is known as 'floating'. Shoulder = midshaft clavicle and neck of the glenoid. This usually indicates a high energy injury and means it is inherently unstable and requires surgical fixation.

Humeral Fractures

Humeral fractures are generally high energy injuries in the young or low energy injuries in elderly patients sustaining a fall.

- Proximal: Most can be managed conservatively in a collar and cuff which allows the weight of the hanging arm to traction the fracture. These can be discharged with follow up in fracture clinic. Comminuted fractures involving the humeral head may require surgical fixation or arthroplasty.
- Mid shaft: Rarely require surgery, coaptation splinting and functional brace are the mainstay of management for two-part mid-shaft fractures. ED should have humeral braces/splints.
- Distal: These are commonly intra-articular fractures and tend to be unstable injuries. Conservative management may be indicated for two-part non-displaced fractures, but operative intervention is usually required.

It is important to use your system of radiograph review and not be distracted by the obvious injury – **do not miss a fracture dislocation of the proximal humerus.**

Upper limb dislocations

- Hand dislocations will be covered in chapter 6.
- Shoulder – XRs are important to determine whether the dislocation is anterior or posterior (Figure 4a and b). Posterior dislocations are rare (<5%) but should be considered particularly for those with fits or electric shocks. Watch out for humeral fractures or bony lesions such as Bankart or Hill Sachs deformities (Figure 4c). We wouldn't advise inexperienced SHOs attempt relocation.
- Sternoclavicular joint dislocations are an unusual but important injury to identify. Posterior dislocations can cause airway compromise and vascular injury and should therefore be discussed with seniors for guidance on further management.

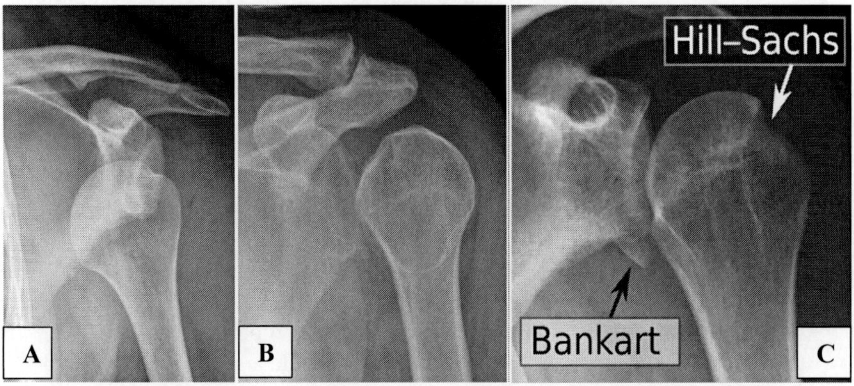

Figure 4. *Demonstrates appearances on AP shoulder radiographs. A) Anterior shoulder dislocation; B) Posterior shoulder dislocation; C) Hill-Sachs and Bankart lesions post reduction of a different shoulder (Wikipedia, 2019).*

Section 6: Lower-limb

Neck of Femur Fractures

Neck of femur fractures are possibly the commonest fractures you will see and a group which will likely require the most attention as they require admission, often with a prolonged hospital stay. Most hospitals have a hip fracture pathway as there are strict criteria to be met which earn the hospitals money – if you can meet these criteria then you will be a friend to the team. Requirements to be aware of include - AMTS, regional block, and preparations for surgery within 36 hours – so NBM for a suitable theatre slot with IV fluids and hold anticoagulation where applicable on admission as per hospital policies. It is often necessary, and in many hospitals part of the protocol, to involve the medical team (ortho-geriatrics in hours and acute medical team out of hours). Don't be afraid to get the medical team involved out of hours. If the patient is not properly worked up pre-theatre, it may delay their operation. These patients typically have multiple comorbidities and polypharmacy including anticoagulants – **familiarise yourself with the hospital's guidelines to reduce the risk of delaying surgery**.

A neck of femur fracture in a young patient is an orthopaedic emergency and requires prompt management to attempt to reduce the risk of avascular necrosis. Many centres will list these first on the trauma list the following morning but the decision not to take these to theatre out of hours rests with a senior orthopod – **call your registrar!**

> **TIP** – if the patient has a history of malignancy – request long leg femur views

These patients invariably require surgery, so a cannula and bloods including Group and Save are mandatory. An ECG, CXR and regional block should also be performed by ED.

Extracapsular fractures usually require fixation with a Dynamic Hip Screw or an Intramedullary nail – this is often centre dependent. Subtrochanteric or reverse oblique fractures usually require a nail and are often pathological (Figure 5).

Figure 5. *Neck of femur fracture classifications.*
See colour centrefold for this image.

NICE guidance dictates that for displaced intracapsular fractures, you should offer total hip replacement rather than hemiarthroplasty to patients who:

1. Were able to walk independently outdoors with no more than the use of a stick AND
2. Are not cognitively impaired AND
3. Are medically fit for anaesthesia and the procedure

Mid-shaft Femur fractures should be managed with skin traction on the ward prior to definitive surgery to improve pain and reduce bleeding.

Ankle fractures

Ankle fractures where dislocation has occurred require satisfactory reduction before a patient can go home. To establish if dislocated, AP (mortise view) and lateral XRs are required. Simply look to see if the Talus is appropriately below the tibia on the mortise view, the trick is to look for a uniform gap around the talus (see diagram).

When examining an ankle, assess the patient's ability to weight bear, look for bruising and swelling, palpate for tenderness along the whole length of the fibula and the medial and lateral malleoli. Examine foot pulses and distal sensation. Palpate for tenderness in the midfoot and hindfoot to identify distal injury.

Figure 6. *Ankle fracture patterns and associated ligamentous injuries.*
See colour centrefold for this image.

Ankle fractures are usually a twisting force, involving damage to bones and ligaments of the ankle. The Weber Classification gives an indication of the stability of the ankle (Figure 6). Weber A fractures can usually be managed conservatively. Weber C fractures usually require surgery. Weber B fractures require surgery if there are other markers of instability (Figure 6).

An interosseous syndesmotic injury can be seen as decreased tibiofibular overlap (Figure 7). This determines whether the ankle can displace laterally. The deep deltoid ligament on the medial side also prevents antero-medial displacement and can be assessed by looking for increased medial clear space on the mortise view aka Talar shift (Figure 8) and/or a fractured medial malleolus.

Figure 7. *AP Radiography of a bimalleolar right ankle fracture. blue arrow=tailor shift, orange = increased medial clear space, green=tib/fib overlap, measured 1cm above the joint line (<5mm is abnormal on mortice view XR) (Wikipedia, 2019).*
See colour centrefold for this image.

The lateral XR is also important to look for posterior malleolus fractures. If no fibular fracture is seen at the ankle, a full length/proximal tibia XR should be requested to find a high fibular fracture (Maisonneuve fracture).

Non-operative treatment includes below knee back slab or a walking boot if the injury is stable. If the ankle cannot be reduced by ED or the SHO then they should call their registrar overnight if significant displacement as it is bad for soft tissues/swelling to leave dislocated for too long. This may involve Manipulation Under Anaesthetic (MUA) and casting or application of a frame. This rarely happens overnight but is worth calling the registrar about if you are unsure.

Surgery involves open reduction and internal fixation depending on the fracture pattern. If the fracture has been reduced then the patient can be sent home that evening with instructions to remain non-weight bearing with strict elevation and be contacted by the trauma coordinator the following morning. It is advisable for them to be starved until called the next day in case there is theatre space. Where possible, definitive surgery is performed when swelling has reduced enough to enable closure over the lateral malleolus (skin should start wrinkling).

Lisfranc Injuries

Are injuries disrupting the tarso-metatarsal joint, which may include a fracture or be purely ligamentous. These are easily missed and can go on to cause progressive pain and deformity.

Patients usually present with significant pain, unable to weight bear, significant swelling, and plantar bruising. They have tenderness over the tarsometatarsal joints.

AP, lateral, oblique and stress XRs are required (figure 8). In the acute setting weight bearing views may be too painful. CT is frequently helpful. These injuries require discussion with a senior and usually necessitate surgical management.

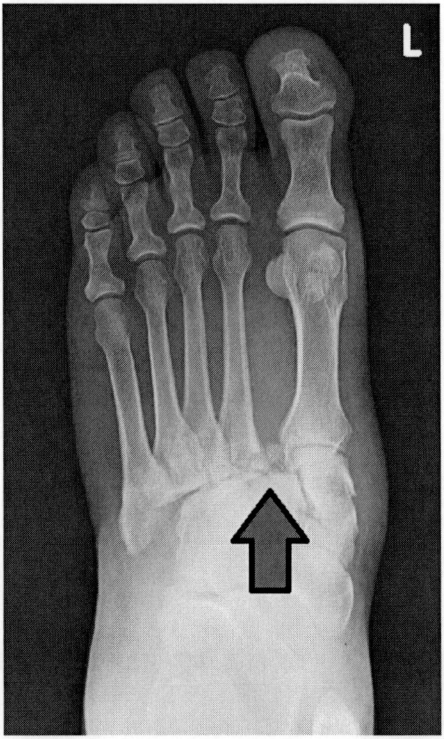

Figure 8. *AP Radiograph of the left foot showing a LisFranc Injury with increased gap and evidence of a bony fracture fragment between the 1st and 2nd ray (Wikipedia, 2019).*

Tibia/ Fibular fractures

Tibial plateau fractures – Look for a split and/or depressed section of bone in the tibial plateau on AP and lateral radiographs of the knee. A CT scan is often required to delineate the nature of the fracture and to plan for surgery. These patients should be discussed with the registrar and usually require admission. For minimally displaced fractures, a hinged knee brace and partial weight bearing for 8-12 weeks may be appropriate. A key sign not to miss is a lipohaemarthrosis on the lateral knee radiograph – this may signify a minimally displaced fracture.

Tibial shaft fractures – Are often either low energy, twisting injuries or high energy impact injuries. AP and lateral XRs are required to assess the fracture. Associated soft tissue injuries are common with high energy injuries. The level of treatment required depends on the severity of the injury and contamination. It is also vital to check for signs of compartment syndrome (see section 10) as high energy tibial fractures are at particularly high risk.

Lower limb dislocations

As with all dislocations, remember to assess NV status pre and post reduction.

- Hip – Native hip dislocation is a high energy injury and an orthopaedic emergency, you should involve your registrar from the outset.
    - Prosthetic hip dislocation – look at imaging to assess whether posterior or anterior and traction and rotate accordingly. If you are unable to reduce the hip, surgical relocation may be required.
- Knee – This is an orthopaedic emergency indicating a high energy injury, with significant risk of vascular injury or nerve damage. **Inform your registrar from the outset** and do not send these patients home overnight as they require neurovascular and compartment observations. Urgent reduction is required and a CT angiogram (CTA) likely indicated to demonstrate any vascular injury. It may be appropriate for CTA to wait until the morning if admitted overnight but this should be discussed with the registrar.
- Ankle –With inline traction the deforming force should be exaggerated and then reversed to reduce the fracture. It is important that the ankle is cast in neutral (often left in plantar flexion).

Section 7: Pelvic Fractures

Pubic rami fractures in isolation are a common result of a fall in the frail elderly. Be sure to also palpate the sacrum and sacro-iliac joints to assess for any tenderness. Treatment involves analgesia and physiotherapy as well as orthogeriatric input. They may not be able to mobilise following the fall and therefore occult neck of femur fracture may need to be ruled out.

More complex pelvic fractures, particularly following high energy injuries require input from a senior early as they have the potential to bleed significantly and may need to be managed in a specialist centre.

Basic ATLS principles are important. Do not 'spring' the pelvis. If a fracture is identified in a resus scenario, apply a pelvic binder if not already in situ. If a binder is not available use a bed-sheet. This should be applied at the level of the greater trochanters. You should also tie the ankles/feet together (internal rotation) to further reduce intra-pelvic volume. Remember to check distal neurovascular status. Check for blood at the urethral meatus. Check the perineum and rectum for signs of an open injury.

Section 8: Septic joints

The hot swollen joint is a common orthopaedic referral.

History

Ask about fevers, joint pain, are they moving the joint or can they weight bear on it? Are they immunocompromised (e.g. diabetes steroids, immunosuppressant medications)? Are they an intravenous drug user? Have they had recent surgery? Do they have a past medical history of arthritis or including gout? Have they got infection/cellultis elsewhere? Are other joints involved?

Examination

Examine for erythema, joint effusion, tenderness and range of motion. If there is a full pain free range of motion, septic arthritis is unlikely. Look for possible sources of infection such as skin wounds. Beware olecranon bursitis / pre-patella bursitis that is commonly mistaken for septic arthritis – aspirating through this could introduce infection into the joint. If in doubt consult your registrar.

Investigations

Obtain X-rays – minimum two views, blood tests (including WCC, and CRP). If infection in a native joint is suspected, discuss with your registrar, who may ask you to take an aspirate and send for urgent M,C+S, gram stain and crystals. It is important that antibiotics are not started prior to aspiration

unless the patient is unwell. This usually requires a call to the lab to make them aware. This should be done overnight and the results chased.
Top tip – micro samples have a habit of going astray in the middle of the night. Keep an extra "spare" sample of the fluid until you know that it is safely in the lab. Neither you nor the patient will relish a second aspirate.

Differential diagnoses to consider

- Flare of OA (remember loss of joint space, subchondral sclerosis, osteophytes and cysts)
- Gout and pseudogout (look for meniscal chondrocalcinosis)
- Charcot foot
- Cellulitis
- Pre-patellar bursitis.

A thorough past medical history helps when considering these differentials. Truly septic joints should be managed with antibiotics and urgent washout (arthroscopic or open) or serial aspirations, depending on the joint and the patient profile. IV antibiotics should be started as soon as possible **after** the aspirate. If left untreated, bacteria rapidly destroy the joint cartilage. Staph aureus counts for over 50% of cases.

If the aspirate is in keeping with septic arthritis, you should call the registrar. If the joint in question is prosthetic, the aspiration should be performed in theatre and you should involve your registrar early even overnight.

Section 9: Osteomyelitis

Patients may present very differently according to the nature and location of the infection. They often present with fevers, tachycardia and may have pain. They may have known chronic osteomyelitis eg in a diabetic foot infection.

Common causes:

- Trauma – particularly with open fractures or devitalised tissue
- Post-surgery – metalwork increases the risk
- Haematogenous spread – from other sites of infection
- Diabetes
- Soft tissue compromise (pressure sores, ulcers)

Investigations:

- Start with an XRay on admission.
- Routine bloods including FBC and CRP.
- MRI scans are often helpful to identify or delineate the extent of osteomyelitis but are unlikely to be necessary overnight.

Management:

- In the acute setting admission depends on how unwell the patient is.
- Long term antibiotics is often the mainstay of treatment.
- Some cases require surgical debridement and referral to a tertiary centre.

Section 10: Compartment Syndrome

The orthopaedic SHO on call will often be called to see a patient with suspected compartment syndrome. This can occur anywhere in the body where muscles are grouped together in a fascial compartment including the lower leg, thigh, hand, forearm, foot, buttock, paraspinal muscles and abdomen. 69% of compartment syndrome cases are due to a fracture (Orthobullets, 2016) but it may also be seen with crush injuries (including intra-operative positioning), burns, post-op or due to tight dressings.

Take a history from the patient. The cardinal symptom is **severe pain despite adequate (opiate) analgesia**. On examination you may be able to feel how tight the compartment is and test for pain on passive stretching. Paraesthesia, paralysis and pulselessness are late signs and should not be waited for to make a diagnosis. If compartment syndrome is suspected, split any casts, bandages or dressings. **Every** patient in whom compartment syndrome is suspected should be escalated with the senior team members immediately and prepared for theatre. In an unconscious or unreliable patient, compartment pressures may be taken (compartment syndrome diagnosed as absolute pressure over 30mmHg or if diastolic BP – compartment pressure = <30mmHg).

Section 11: Spinal injuries

Spinal injuries can be intimidating to a cross covering SHO and if in any doubt speak to your registrar. Cases requiring surgery may need urgent referral to a tertiary centre.

C-spine

Patients with C-spine injuries may arrive in a collar with blocks. ATLS management is essential on initial presentation. If there is a high energy mechanism or the patient is complaining of neck pain, pain on moving their neck, or has c-spine tenderness, a CT cervical spine should be performed to establish any bony injury. This is often already performed by ED according to Canadian C-spine, NICE and BOAST 2 Guidelines (Stiell et al. 2001, NICE 2019, BOAST 2 2008). C-spine fractures may be missed in the acute trauma scenario, particularly in the presence of multi-trauma or unconscious/sedated patients.

A careful neurological exam should be performed, using an American Spinal Injuries Association (ASIA) chart is a helpful reminder and an excellent way of recording your findings – google a PDF version, print out and fill in.

Removal of the collar can only be performed without imaging if:

- The patient is awake, alert, not intoxicated AND
- Has no neck tenderness, painful neck movements or neurologic defects AND
- Has no distracting injuries (NICE, 2019 and BOAST 2, 2008)

Thoracic spine

Fractures of T2-T10 are rare due to the rib cage providing relative stability. Fracture patterns and principles of management of fractures in this region do follow those of the lumbar spine below.

Thoracolumbar spine

- Burst fractures:
    - Commonly occur in thoracolumbar region T11-L2 due to axial trauma causing fracture at the fulcrum

below the relatively rigid thoracic spine. These can be unstable because both anterior and middle columns can be involved (Figure 10).
- Fragments of the vertebral body can burst backwards into the spinal cord causing neurological damage.
- Be sure to get XRs of the entire spine. In 20% of cases there may be a fracture at another level. On AP a burst fracture may be seen as widening of the pedicles, on the lateral, look for deformity in the lines (Figure 10) or fragments of retropulsed bone.
- If there is bony deformity or neurological change, obtain a CT. MRI scans show ligamentous damage or cord/nerve root injury. Discuss any neurological injury with seniors immediately. These patients should be on bed rest and log rolled. You should not be independently providing an opinion on stability.
- Patients who are neurologically intact or have a stable fracture pattern (worth discussing this with a senior) can be managed in a TLSO (Thoracic Lumbar Sacral Orthosis) brace. Otherwise surgery may be required for decompression and spinal stabilisation.

- Osteoporotic compression fracture
    - Again, take a thorough history, examination and XRs of the entire spine (20% have a further fracture).
    - Consider primary malignancy (e.g. myeloma) or metastatic disease as an underlying cause in the young or for fractures above T5
    - These fractures are usually stable, neurologically intact and can be managed conservatively with analgesia.

- Fracture/dislocation (Chance fracture)
    - These are high energy injuries, from rapid deceleration/hyperflexion, causing compression of the anterior column and distraction of the posterior column, frequently associated with neurological injury.
    - These fractures have a high incidence of associated intra-abdominal injury – **get early general surgical input**

- Lateral radiograph or CT scan may show an acute fracture, exaggerated kyphosis or a step. MRI scans are often also required to demonstrate ligamentous stability and cord involvement.

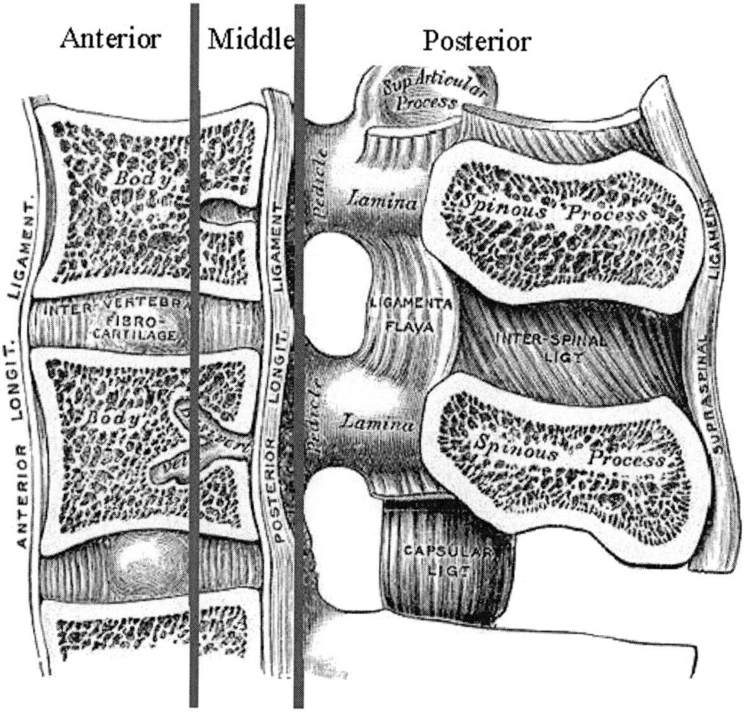

Figure 9. *Diagrammatic section of a sagittal section through the lumbar spine illustrating the position of the three spinal columns. (Edited image from Gray's anatomy of the human body)*

Figure 10. *Lateral XR of the Cervical spine, with each vertebrae numbered and lines to demonstrate: anterior vertebral line (blue), posterior vertebral line (yellow), spino-laminar line (red), posterior spinous line (green) (Wikipedia, 2019).*
See colour centrefold for this image.

Lumbar disc herniation – is a common cause of back pain presenting to the ED department. If there is no associated acute neurology, they should be managed with analgesia, initial rest followed by progressive activity and in 90% symptoms will resolve (Orthobullets, 2019).

Cauda equina – any new/increased back pain with any new bladder/bowel symptoms/saddle anaesthesia/sexual dysfunction/loss of power or altered sensation symptoms should be discussed with a senior and urgent MRI likely required. Document a full neurological examination including perianal pinprick sensation and digital rectal examination including "squeeze". Document post-void residual bladder scan. If the patient is catheterised then document sensation from a 'catheter tug' (GENTLE traction on the catheter). Suspected cauda equina syndrome mandates discussion with your registrar and a request for an urgent MRI scan at any time of day. If proven on an MRI scan, urgent surgical decompression is often required to prevent permanent neurology.

Section 12: Paediatric orthopaedics

You may commonly get asked to review a limping child or a child with a painful hip or knee. Take a full history and examine the patient. Remember to examine the joint above and below. Look at the plantar aspect of the foot for tenderness or injury, assess joints as you would for any septic arthritis and note symmetry of movement. Remember to carefully document everything and have a high index of suspicion for non- accidental injury. If there are any concerns you should consult with the on-call paediatric team to arrange admission (hospital is a place of safety) and follow your trust guidance.

For paediatric fractures, the Salter Harris classification is commonly used and helpful to be familiar with. These are paediatric fractures involving the physis (growth plate) and are commonly seen injuries (Figure 11).

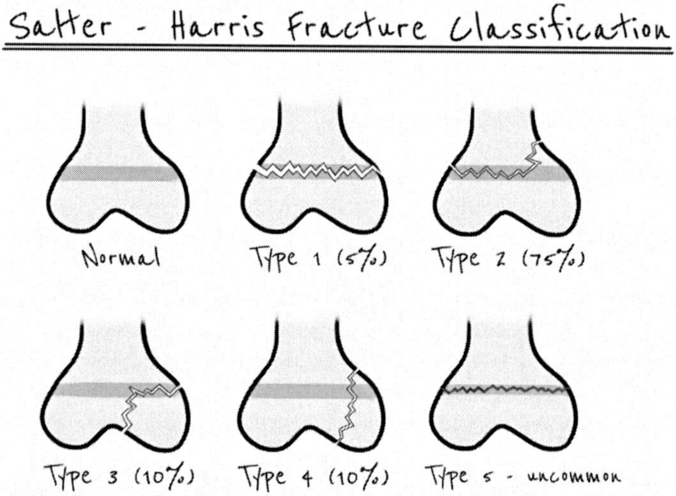

Figure 11. *Diagram illustrating the Salter Harris classification for fractures involving the epiphysis of long bones.*

Septic hip

History:

- Depending on age, the child may be lethargic and dehydrated (not wetting nappies).

Kocher's criteria for septic hip are a good guide (Kocher, Zurakowshi and Kasser, 1999):

-
    - Temp > 38.5 C
    - Unable to bear weight
    - WCC > 12/CRP > 20/ESR>40
- Have they had any hip problems in the past? Have they got infection elsewhere? Any recent illness? (transient synovitis)

Examination:

- A septic hip is painful

- Pain on active and passive movement

Investigations:

- Obtain bloods including WCC, ESR and CRP.
- You may see an effusion on a hip XR as a laterally displaced femoral head in the acetabulum. (this is a subtle sign)

If septic hip is suspected, this should be discussed with your registrar immediately and ultrasound guided hip aspiration may give you a diagnosis.

Management:

This involves early IV antibiotics (ideally after aspirate) and open washout in theatre or repeated aspiration to dryness. Do not start antibitioics without discussion with a senior unless the patient is unwell.

Disorders of the hip

Remember that pain in the thigh/knee can almost be considered to originate from the hip until proven otherwise. Here we run through a few of the more common paediatric hip problems.

- Developmental dysplasia of the hip:
    - Presents at <2 years (should be picked up as newborn in the UK). This should be managed in the outpatient setting.
    - Examination demonstrated limited hip abduction and leg length discrepancy with trendelenberg gait and toe walking once ambulant age.
    - Imaging involves Ultrasound scanning (USS) if <4 months or XRay if >4 months old.
    - Treatment as a newborn is usually with closed reduction and a Pavlik Harness.

- Perthes' disease:
    - Presents at 4-8 years.
    - 5 Male : 1 Female (Orthobullets, 2018)
    - 12% are bilateral.
    - The onset of the disease is rather insidious, with a limp and/or intermittent groin/knee pain.

- AP and frog/leg lateral XRays are required for diagnosis.
- Management is usually as an outpatient and can be non-operative with anti-inflammatories, restricted weight bearing and physiotherapy or operative for more advanced disease.

- Slipped Upper femoral Epiphysis:
  - Presents as 10-16 years.
  - 2 Male: 1.4 Female. Specific ethnicities include African American, pacific island, Latino (Orthobullets, 2018)
  - Obesity and endocrine abnormalities are risk factors.
  - Patients usually present with groin or knee pain or a limp.
  - AP and frog-lateral XRs are required and you may see the femoral epiphysis 'slipping off' the metaphysis. Look for asymmetry in the XRays and review 'klein's lines' – the line normally intersects the epiphysis (Figure 12). These signs can be subtle so if you are unsure consult a senior or admit for bed rest prior to discussion in the morning.
  - This requires discussion with the registrar and admission for bed rest. Treatment is with percutaneous fixation in-situ using one or two cannulated screws to either the affected side or both sides – this remains controversial.

Figure 12. *Frog leg lateral radiograph of paediatric left hip. Klein's line drawn along superior aspect of femoral neck – A slipped upper femoral epiphysis is evident as the line does not intersect the femoral head. (Annotated original image from, Wikipedia, 2019)*
See colour centrefold for this image.

Paediatric trauma

Supracondylar elbow fractures are common presentation, often after a fall onto an outstretched hand. Your examination must test the neurovascular status:

- Particular attention to Anterior Interosseous Nerve (branch of median) with the 'OK sign' demonstrating intact flexor pollicis longus.
- Assessing all nerves can be difficult with kids an easy way is – OK sign *(Anterior Interosseous Nerve -from Median)*, rock, paper *(from rock to paper = Radial)*, scissors *(Ulnar)*.

- You should palpate the radial artery and assess capillary refill time.

Investigations:

- AP and lateral XRs are required. Look at the anterior humeral and radio-capitellar lines to identify displacement (Figure 13a).
- A line through the radius should bisect the capitellum (this is very important and commonly missed) and a line down the anterior aspect of the humerus should travel through the anterior 1/3 of the trochlear. The anterior and posterior fat pads can also be seen on XRay as a sign of elbow injury (figure 13b).

Figure 13. *a) Lateral radiograph of an uninjured skeletally immature elbow. Red = radiocapitellar line, blue = anterior humeral line b) Lateral radiography of a skeletally mature elbow, demonstrating anterior and posterior fat pad signs. (Annotated original image from, Wikipedia, 2019)*
See colour centrefold for this image.

Management:

- If there is any neurovascular disturbance urgent manipulation or surgery is required.
- Even if neurovascularly intact, children with these fractures should be discussed with seniors as they often require surgery. If seen overnight they should usually be admitted but at least discussed with a senior.
- They should be cast in a position of comfort prior to surgery.

References

British Orthopaedic Association Standards for Trauma, 2008 http://www.necn.nhs.uk/wp-content/uploads/2014/05/BOAST-2.pdf

British Orthopaedic Association Standards for Trauma, 2017. https://www.boa.ac.uk/wp-content/uploads/2017/12/BOAST-Open-Fractures.pdf

Gustilo RB, Anderson JT. Prevention of infection in the treatment of one thousand and twenty-five open fractures of long bones. J Bone Joint Surg Am 1976;58:453-8

https://commons.wikimedia.org/wiki/File:Dislocated_shoulder_X-ray_10.png#filelinks. Uploaded by User 'Hellerhoff' with creative commons license held at: https://creativecommons.org/licenses/by-sa/3.0/deed.en

https://en.wikipedia.org/wiki/Cervical_vertebrae#/media/File:HWS_seitlich_Annotation.jpg Uploaded by user Hellerhoff with creative commons license held at: https://creativecommons.org/licenses/by-sa/3.0/deed.en

https://en.wikipedia.org/wiki/Fat_pad_sign#/media/File:Fettpolsterzeichen_pathologisch_Ellenbogen.png Uploaded by user Hellerhoff with creative commons license held at: https://creativecommons.org/licenses/by-sa/3.0/deed.en

https://en.wikipedia.org/wiki/Humeroradial_joint#/media/File:Radiocapitellar_line_-_normal.jpg Uploaded by user Mikael Häggström with creative commons license held at: https://creativecommons.org/licenses/by-sa/4.0/deed.en

https://en.wikipedia.org/wiki/Ligamenta_flava#/media/File:Gray301.png Uploaded by user Dzenanz with license in the public domain in its country of origin and other countries and areas where the copyright term is the author's life plus 100 years or less.

https://en.wikipedia.org/wiki/Lisfranc_injury#/media/File:LisFrancArrow.png. Uploaded by user James Heilman, MD with creative commons license held at: https://creativecommons.org/licenses/by-sa/4.0/deed.en

https://en.wikipedia.org/wiki/Scaphoid_bone#/media/File:Scaphoidfraktur_1_pfeil.jpg. Uploaded by User 'Sjoehest' with creative commons license held at: https://creativecommons.org/licenses/by-sa/3.0/deed.en

https://en.wikipedia.org/wiki/Slipped_capital_femoral_epiphysis#/media/File:SCFE_FROG_B%26W.jpg released into the public domain by its author, Mikir at English Wikipedia

https://en.wikipedia.org/wiki/Trimalleolar_fracture#/media/File:Trimalleolar_Ankle_Fracture_Xray_shown_before_surgery_and_after_surgery.png Uploaded by User Chaim Mintz with creative commons license held at: https://creativecommons.org/licenses/by-sa/3.0/deed.en

https://upload.wikimedia.org/wikipedia/commons/6/6f/PchancefracCT.png. Uploaded by User James Heilman, MD with creative commons license held at: https://creativecommons.org/licenses/by-sa/3.0/deed.en

https://upload.wikimedia.org/wikipedia/commons/b/be/Lightbulb_sign_-_posterior_shoulder_dislocation_Roe_vor_und_nach_Reposition_001.jpg. Uploaded by User 'Hellerhoff' with creative commons license held at: https://creativecommons.org/licenses/by-sa/3.0/deed.en

https://upload.wikimedia.org/wikipedia/commons/e/e3/Shoulder_dislocation_with_Bankart_and_Hill-Sachs_lesion%2C_before_and_after_ reduction.jpg Uploaded by User 'Mikael Häggström' with creative commons license held at: https://creativecommons.org/licenses/by-sa/3.0/deed.en

Kocher MS, Zurakowski D, Kasser JR (1999). "Differentiating between septic arthritis and transient synovitis of the hip in children: an evidence-based clinical prediction algorithm". J Bone Joint Surg Am. 81(12): 1662–70. doi:10.2106/00004623-199912000-00002. PMID 10608376.

Loder RT, Skopelja EN. The epidemiology and demographics of slipped capital femoral epiphysis. ISRN Orthop. 2011:486512

Mazloumi SM, Ebrahimzadeh MH, Kachooei AR. Evolution in diagnosis and treatment of Legg-Calve-Perthes disease. Arch Bone Jt Surg. 2014;2(2):86–92.

National Institute For Clinical Excellence, 2019 https://pathways.nice.org.uk/pathways/head-injury/investigation-for-injuries-to-the-cervical-spine-in-patients-with-head-injury#content=view-node%3Anodes-risk-factors-indicating-ct-cervical-spine-scan-within-1-hour-in-adults

Stiell IG, et al. The Canadian C-spine rule for radiography in alert and stable trauma patients. JAMA. 2001 Oct 17; 286 (15): 1841-8

CHAPTER 8

UROLOGY

JOHN PASCOE & JENNIFER MARTIN

Abstract
Section 1 – Introduction
Section 2 – The Acute Scrotum
Section 3 – Renal colic
Section 4 – Urinary retention & The Difficult Catheter
Section 5 – Haematuria
Section 6 – Foreskin Emergencies
Section 7 – Urological Trauma
Section 8 – Priapism
Section 9 – Infections
Simple
Complicated
Pyelonephritis
Fournier's Gangrene

Abstract

This chapter is designed to provide a guide for junior doctor's cross-covering urology as well as providing a solid framework to approach the common indicative presentations you may encounter including: the acute scrotum, renal colic, urinary retention, catheter complications, haematuria, foreskin emergencies, priapism, urological trauma and urological infections This will allow you to provide safe care with confidence whilst on-call. We also provide helpful tips and tricks when performing practical procedures and guidance on further reading for those looking for greater detail.

Section 1: Introduction

Most junior doctors will have a rotation through surgery throughout postgraduate training. Some may have the luxury of a urology-focussed job, whilst some may only see it in a cross-cover capacity. The cross-cover role is to start immediate management as well as recognise emergencies and know when to seek help. When you become more confident you should be able to safely discharge patients and arrange appropriate follow up.

This chapter is designed to provide a guide for junior doctors cross covering urology as well as to have a solid framework to approach the common indicative presentations you may encounter. Whilst it will provide references for further reading to expand your knowledge base, it does not intend to negotiate the specifics of paediatric urology, urinary incontinence or the complex penoplasty.

Red Flags: These are the features of an indicative presentation that point toward a more serious pathology that might require urgent investigation and intervention. In the presence of these red flags early urology opinion should be sought.

This chapter will hopefully make your time on urology cross cover more enjoyable and provide a safer environment for your patients.

Section 2: The Acute Scrotum

"Hi Doctor, I'm worried this boy has a testicular torsion" – the 1am phone call from the ED SHO

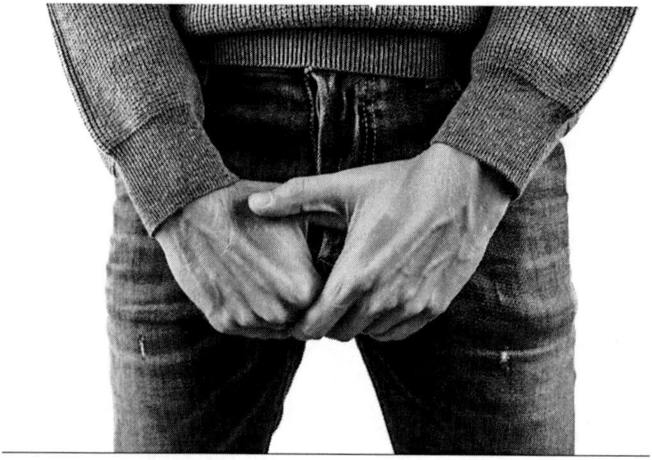

Figure 1 – *Testicular pain (Pixabay 2017)*

This is testicular torsion until proven otherwise.

Questions to ask at the time of referral?

- How old is the patient?
- When did the pain come on?
- History of testicular problems before?
- Nausea/Vomiting?
- Trauma?
- What does the scrotum look like?
- When did they last eat & drink? Please keep them nil-by-mouth (NBM)

Testicular torsion definition:

- An acute urological emergency characterised by a twisting of the spermatic cord causing ischaemia
- Without prompt action the loss of blood flow to the testicle can result in the loss of the testicle due to irreversible ischaemia (figure 2).

Figure 2. *An animal demonstration comparing testicular torsion. Normal, Left & Torted, Right.* (Wikipedia 2007)
See colour centrefold for this image.

Red Flags:

As the urology SHO you will be referred many patients with testicular pain as suspected testicular torsion, fortunately the numbers that actually are torsion will be small. However, these may still warrant surgical exploration. The role of the cross-cover doctor is the assume torsion till convinced otherwise. The following "red flags" are alerts that should make you more concerned of a possible torsion.

- Age <25
    - Due to the anatomical aetiology of testicular torsion it is unusual in those over the age of 25.
    - Peak incidence is at puberty between 13-16 years
    - Can occur in utero and in neonates, though this is fortunately rare
- A short history of severe, acute unilateral testicular pain
- Precipitating history of intermittent similar pains that resolve and return
    - Maybe indicative of intermittent torsion and warrant exploration
- Nausea +/- vomiting
- Precipitating trauma
- Abnormal appearance of the testicle:
    - Swelling & erythema
    - High-riding testicle
    - Bell-clapper testicle
    - In late presentations, there may be discolouration of the skin on the affected side
    - Loss of the cremasteric reflex

Differential	Differentiating features
Epididymo-orchitis	• Usually co-exists with urinary tract infection/Sexually transmitted infection • Phren's sign (**e**levation **e**ases **e**pididymitis) • Less acute onset • Typically affects older population • Ultrasound **may** prove diagnostic
Torted hydatid of Morgagni (Testicular appendage)	• In the eyes of an experienced clinician a "blue dot" may be visible • Less acute onset
Idiopathic scrotal oedema	• An acute self-limiting condition of oedema of the skin & dartos layers of the scrotum typically affecting young boys. • Experienced sonographers may be able to pick up this condition on ultrasound by identifying the 'fountain sign' • Surgical exploration is not necessary in this group unless another diagnosis is suspected
Testicular tumour	• More commonly painless • Ultrasound will show presence of tumour
Renal Colic	• Pain from renal colic can refer to the tip of the penis and testicle • The features of renal colic are more predominantly flank/groin pain & microscopic haematuria. • CT-KUB will confirm diagnosis
Scrotal abscess	• Acutely tender, but fluctuant scrotal mass palpable • Patient may show signs of systemic infection • Ultrasound will show the presence of an abscess
Hydrocele	• Transilluminates light easily • Usually not painful • Diagnosed on ultrasound
Varicocele	• Dragging pain, less acute • Diagnosed clinically, but can be demonstrated on ultrasound
Scrotal Haematoma	• Usually a clear history of trauma • Ultrasound will confirm presence of haematoma and can show evidence of potential testicular rupture
Mumps	• The vast majority of patients with mumps have enlarged parotid glands • Patient's will typically describe bilateral scrotal pain and swelling • Whilst scrotal swelling may occur in mumps, the systemic features of mumps make the diagnosis clearer

Table 1. *Differential diagnosis for testicular torsion*

Differential Diagnosis

Only a small number of males presenting with testicular pain will actually have testicular torsion and the differential diagnosis can be broad (table 1).

Investigating the acute scrotum

If there is a high clinical suspicion for testicular torsion – do not waste time with investigations, proceed to theatre. If suspicion is low or other differentials more likely, certain investigations may aid diagnosis & further treatment.

Bedside:

- Urine dipstick
- Urine for microscopy, cultures & sensitivity

Blood tests:

- Inflammatory markers
- Blood cultures if patient showing signs of sepsis

Imaging:

- Ultrasound testes +/- Doppler
    - In cases of testicular pain with a low or unclear clinical suspicion of torsion, when available, ultrasound can have a useful role in excluding torsion
    - Sonographer dependent
    - Gold standard investigation for multiple other scrotal pathologies

Treatment of testicular torsion

- Keep patient NBM
- Analgesia
- Discuss with your senior and prepare the patient for theatre
- The surgical approach of scrotal exploration will vary, however if a true torsion is identified and the testicle is viable after untwisting it, then a scrotal orchidopexy is performed with the creation of a dartos pouch. The contralateral testicle should also be repaired to prevent future torsion on that side.

When to wake the boss

If you suspect a testicular torsion – **do not delay**! Discuss with your senior ASAP. It should be noted, that many hospitals do not have urology or urology cover out of hours and the general surgeons are expected to manage testicular torsion; transfer to another hospital with urology cover is not appropriate (figure 3).

As the cross cover doctor your job is to get this patient ready for theatre.

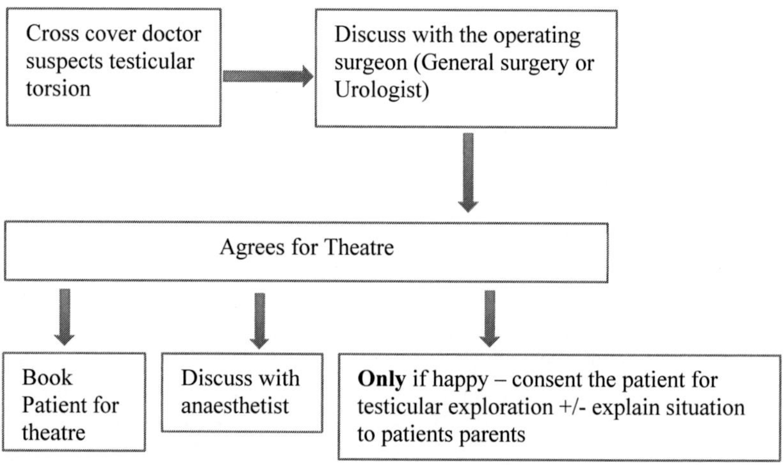

Figure 3. *Management pathways for testicular torsion*

Further reading on the acute scrotum

- A note on consent
    - British Association for Urological Surgeons – Urological Emergencies App
    - A comprehensive overview of urological emergencies and also a source of multiple BAUS approved consent forms that can be printed straight from a phone
- TWIST Score
    - Sheth KR et al. Diagnosing testicular torsion before urological consultation and imaging: Validation of the TWIST score. Journal of Urology, 2016.

    - The TWIST score may be used to help risk stratify patients with suspected torsion further and aid treatment.
- Testicular exploration – operative procedure
    - BMJ Learning Online: Surgical Skills – exploration of the scrotum for testicular torsion.
    - A video run through of the surgical procedure

Section 3: Renal Colic

> *"Hi Doctor, Mr Jones is a 30-year-old farmer screaming from flank pain & there's blood in the urine. Could it be renal colic?"*
> – The nurse practitioner at the local minor injury unit.

The questions the cross-cover doctor should ask at the time of referral?

- Have we ruled out other serious pathologies?
    - Abdominal aortic aneurysms and pancreatitis may present similarly early on.
- Are they septic?
- Have you arranged a NCCT (Non-Contrast Computer Tomography) KUB (kidney, ureter & bladder)? – many urology units will not accept a patient with suspected renal colic unless it has been confirmed on CT
- Have we got blood results? Is there renal function affected?
- Do they have any history of renal/urological disease?
    - Single or transplanted kidney?
    - Chronic kidney disease

Definitions:

- Urolithiasis refers to the precipitation of crystalline calculi along the urinary tract
- Renal colic refers to the intermittent pain caused by the stone within the ureter

Risk factors for renal colic:

- Epidemiology
    - More common in males
    - Peak incidence in age is 30-60

- Congenital:
    - Genetic conditions e.g cystinuria, renal tubular acidosis, medullary sponge kidney
    - Congenital urinary tract obstruction
    - Family history (~25% of cases)

- Acquired:
    - General factors:
        - obesity
        - Sedentary lifestyle
        - High protein intake
        - High salt intake
        - Dehydration
        - Infectious triggers - certain urinary infections promote the formation of staghorn calculi e.g. proteus, klebsiella

    - Diseases associated with stone formation:
        - Hypercalcaemia: e.g. hyperparathyroidism
        - Hyperuricaemia: e.g. Gout
        - Gastro-intestinal diseases causing malabsorptive states: e.g. inflammatory bowel disease
        - Sarcoidosis
        - Spinal cord injury
        - Metabolic syndrome

    - Pharmacological triggers e.g. chemotherapy

    - Anatomical risk factors
        - Horseshoe kidney
        - Vesico-ureteric reflux
        - Calyceal diverticulum
        - PUJ obstruction

Presenting features for renal colic:

- Pain
    - Classical presentation is acute, severe flank pain, typically radiating to the groin, but dependent on the position of the stone can radiate to the lower abdomen, penis, testicle, labia or lower back.

    - This pain can be intermittent (colicky)
    - It should be noted that stones can be present without pain and are found incidentally on unrelated imaging

- Haematuria
    - >80% of patients have microscopic haematuria
    - Frank haematuria may occur but is much rarer
- Nausea & vomiting
- Voiding lower urinary tract symptoms
- Symptoms/Signs of sepsis
    - As a result of an obstructed infected kidney (see below)
    - Stones may also act as a nidus for infection resulting in recurrent urinary tract infections

Red Flags:

The most serious sequela of renal colic is an infected obstructed system. This is where a ureteric stone obstructs the ureter, with infection of the urine developing proximal to it. This infection can cause rapidly evolving sepsis and significant renal impairment. Suspicion of an infected obstructed system requires urgent imaging and definitive management to drain the sepsis. Support from the intensive care team may be required.

- Sepsis
    - Pyrexia/tachycardia/hypotension/tachypnoea
- Impaired renal function
    - Biochemical evidence of renal failure
    - Poor urine output

The presenting features of a ruptured abdominal aortic aneurysm can mimic renal colic in some patients (table 2), it is essential that these patients are appropriately diagnosed in the emergency department. Presenting features might include: a known aneurysm, haemodynamic instability or significant vascular risk factors: age >60, male gender, smoking and history of hypertension, hypercholesterolemia and cardiac abnormalities. If in doubt, obtain imaging.

Differential diagnosis

Differential	Differentiating features
Abdominal Aortic aneurysm	• If there is haemodyamic instability, presence of significant vascular risk factors or a known aneurysm an urgent CT should be used for differentiation
Pancreatitis	• Amylase will be significantly elevated and patient may be profoundly unwell
Appendicitis	• Renal colic can present with similar right lower quadrant pain however repeated examination with or without imaging will aid in differentiation
Musculoskeletal back pain	• In MSK back pain there may be an obvious mechanical trigger, single point tenderness on palpation of the muscles of the back or sciatica related symptoms. Non-contrast CT KUB will show no stones

Table 2. *Differential diagnosis for ureteric colic.*

Investigating renal colic

Bedside:

- Urine dipstick & M,C&S
- Beta hCG (May influence diagnosis & imaging choices if positive)
- FAST scan (Check for obvious AAA)

Blood tests:

- Inflammatory markers
- U&E
- Calcium/magnesium/uric acid/phosphate
    - Once diagnosis confirmed may suggest aetiology behind stone formation

Imaging:

- CTKUB
    - the gold standard for diagnosing ureteric stones
    - Can demonstrate the size of the stone, presence of obstruction & delineate renal tract anatomy
    - Does not require contrast so safe in renal impairment

- Uses radiation so should not be first line in children or pregnancy

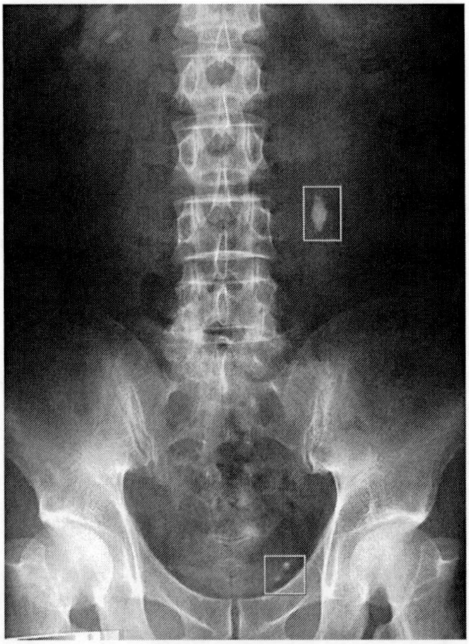

Figure 4. *X Ray KUB of a large left renal stone and distal stones shown within the boxes (Pinterest 2019)*

- USS KUB
  - Can demonstrate presence of hydronephrosis from obstruction & may identify presence of a stone
  - No radiation so first line in children & pregnancy

- XR KUB (figure 4)
  - May show calcium-based stones
  - Should **NOT** be used for diagnosis
  - Can be used after CT confirms diagnosis. If stone is proven to be radio-opaque XR can be used for follow up and avoid the increased radiation dose of repeat CT.

Treatment of renal colic

Initial:

- All patients should receive analgesia
    - Paracetamol & NSAID's - PR diclofenac 150mg (one dose every 16hrs) and IV ketorolac are commonly used
    - Opiate-based medications, such as oral or intravenous morphine may be required
- Antiemetics may be required
- Rehydrate with crystalloids if clinically dehydrated

Definitive:

- 80% of ureteric stones will pass spontaneously.
- Size & position of the stone predict the likelihood of stone passage
- Historically, medical expulsive therapy (MET) has been used to aid expulsion of stones, however evidence supporting this has been inconclusive
- Indications for urgent intervention in stones:
    - Single kidney
    - Uncontrolled pain
    - Septic, obstructed kidney

Outpatient management:

- Extracorporeal Shock Wave Lithotripsy (ESWL)
    - Causes mechanical destruction of stones and assists passage
- Retrograde ureteroscopy +/- stone removal
- Percutaneous nephrolithotomy (PCNL)
- Open/laparoscopic stone removal (rare)

Guidelines on when to admit:

- Stones with infection*
- Suspected stones with significant acute kidney injury*
- Unmanageable pain
- Single/transplanted kidneys*
- Pregnancy
- Those who will have their investigations/management significantly delayed without admission

* These patients are highly likely to need overnight imaging if the diagnosis is suspected

Those who have not had a scan to confirm diagnosis should ideally return in the very near future for a confirmatory scan. Patients with a confirmed diagnosis may require follow up and warrant further discussion.

When to wake the boss

If the patient is demonstrating significant complications secondary to their ureteric stone, such as renal failure or severe sepsis, this will require urgent intervention.

Definitive management in the form of a retrograde ureteric stent or percutaneous nephrostomy (PCN) may be necessary and life-saving to relieve obstruction and drain infection.

Percutaneous nephrostomy

- Performed by interventional radiology
- A tube is placed directly into the renal pelvis to relieve obstruction
- Is usually performed under local anaesthetic
- An antegrade stent can be placed via the nephrostomy catheter at a later date (figure 5)
- Contraindications include: coagulopathy & un-cooperative patients

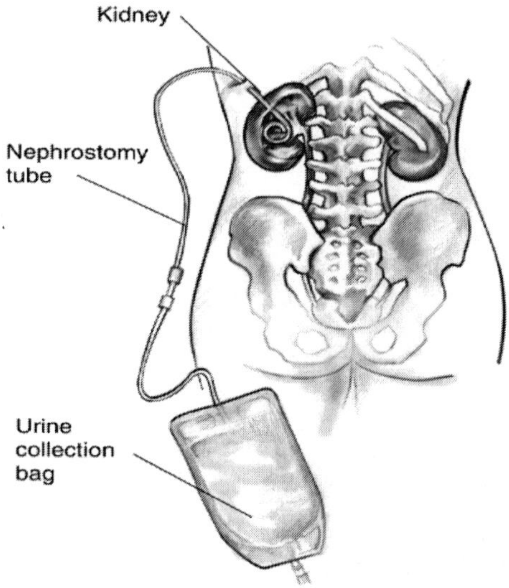

Figure 5. *Illustration of nephrostomy placement. (Wikipedia 2013)*

Retrograde ureteric stenting

- Performed by urology
- Using a rigid cystoscope a ureteric stent is inserted via the affected ureteric orifice and passed down ureter
- This is performed under general anaesthetic
- Concurrent fluoroscopy allows for a retrograde pyelogram and correct positioning
- Stent placement should be recorded appropriately to ensure it is removed promptly
- There are no absolute contraindications, but placement can be difficult in oedematous ureters

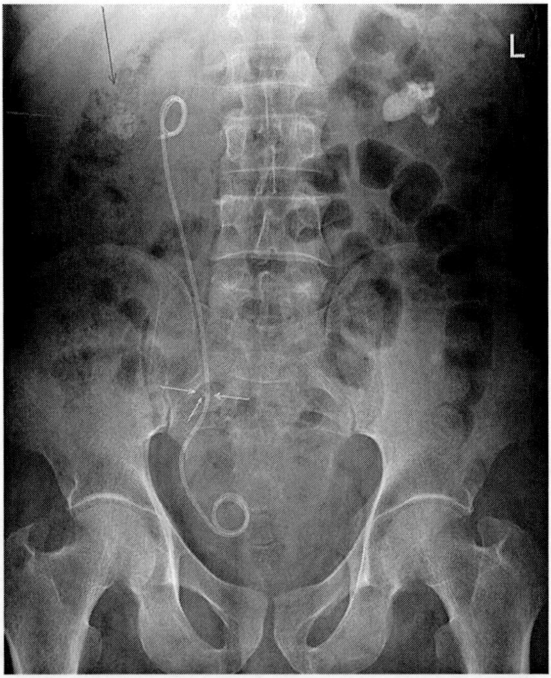

Figure 6. *An XRay KUB with a right JJ ureteric stent, right renal stone (red) & distal ureteric stone (yellow) (Wikipedia 2008)*

Further reading on renal colic

- The evidence regarding medical expulsion therapy
    - Key trials are:
        - Medical expulsive therapy in adults with ureteric colic: a multicentre, randomised, placebo-controlled trial (Pickard et al)
        - Efficacy and Safety of Tamsulosin in Medical Expulsive Therapy for Distal Ureteral Stones with Renal Colic: A Multicenter, Randomized, Double-blind, Placebo-controlled Trial (Zangquen et al)

- Biochemistry of stone formation
    - European association of Urology (EAU) guidelines on urolithiasis

- Percutaneous nephrostomy *vs.* ureteric stenting
    - Key trials are:
        - Optimal method of urgent decompression of the collecting system for obstruction and infection due to ureteral calculi (Pearle et al)
        - Percutaneous nephrostomy versus ureteral stents for diversion of hydronephrosis caused by stones: a prospective, randomized clinical trial (Mokhmalji et al)
        - Emergent ureteric stent vs percutaneous nephrostomy for obstructive urolithiasis with sepsis: patterns of use and outcomes from a 15-year experience (Preminger et al)

Section 4: Urinary Retention & The Difficult Catheter

"Hi Doctor, Mr Jones hasn't passed urine all day and now he's in a lot of pain. I think he's in retention" – The out of hours GP

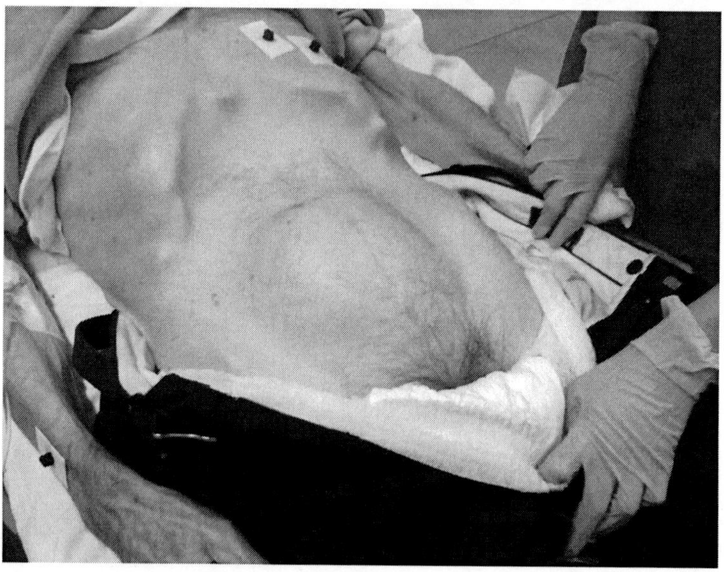

Figure 7. *A visibly distended bladder – a rare sign that may be seen in urinary retention (Wikipedia 2012)*

The questions the cross-cover doctor should ask at the time of referral?

- Has the patient had a bladder scan? Have we actually confirmed retention?
- Are they in pain?
- Have they been catheterised?
    - If the answer is no and the patient is in pain, find a pragmatic approach to get them catheterised ASAP
- Are there any obvious clues pointing towards the aetiology?
- Does the patient have back pain, paraesthesia or saddle anaesthesia?
    - **DO NOT MISS CAUDA EQUINA OR SPINAL CORD COMPRESSION**
- Can we get this patient home? What do we need to do to make this possible?

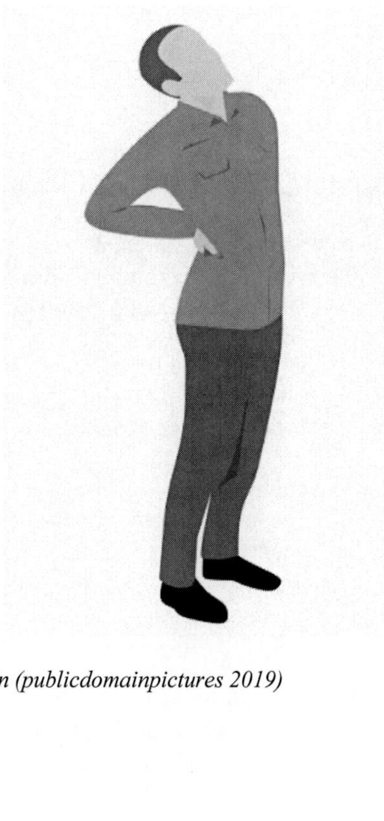

Figure 8. *Flank Pain (publicdomainpictures 2019)*

Definitions

MYTH: "The patient cannot be in retention, they're peeing"

- Acute Urinary Retention:
    - The sudden, painful inability to pass urine
    - Relieved by urethral catheterisation
- Chronic Urinary Retention
    - The inability for the bladder to empty completely, but voiding is still maintained. Can present with lower urinary tract symptoms or nocturnal enuresis.
    - A residual volume of >1L is highly suggestive of chronic retention
    - High pressure chronic retention is diagnosed in those with chronic retention and either hydronephrosis or renal dysfunction

Aetiology

The aetiology of both acute and chronic urinary retention can be subdivided under three main headings:

- Related to bladder outflow obstruction
    - Benign Prostatic Hyperplasia (BPH)
        - BPH is the pathophysiological process causing an increase in size and volume of prostate tissue, which can subsequently cause bladder outlet obstruction in some men the obstruction becomes more pronounced the detrusor muscle of the bladder wall becomes thicker to compensate.
        - However, the thicker bladder wall can become counterintuitive as the new arrangement of muscle fibres eventually become less efficient
    - Infections
        - E.g. prostatitis, balanitis or vulvovaginitis
    - Urethral Stricture/Stenosis
        - Commonly related to recurrent infections or scarring from prior surgery

- Prolapsing pelvic organs
    - Anteriorly the bladder can prolapse into the vagina causing a pinch to the urethra and therefore retention (cystocele).
    - Posteriorly the rectum can also prolapse in to the vagina causing an abnormal position of the urethra and therefore retention (Rectocele).
- Clot retention
    - Patients with significant haematuria can form clots in the static urine. These clots can occlude the urethra.

- Malignancy
    - Prostate, urethral, bladder or gynaecological malignancies can inhibit flow.

- Constipation
    - Faecal loading can commonly cause the rectum to put pressure on the bladder and or urethra inhibiting flow of urine

- Calculi
    - Bladder calculi can obstruct flow of urine

- Neurological
    - The neurological causes or urinary retention are complex and can arise centrally or from peripheral nervous dysfunction.
    - Examples include:
        - Sacral spinal cord injury can result in loss of the detrusor reflex
        - Thoracic cord injury can result in detrusor sphincter dyssynergia (the bladder contracts against a contracted external sphincter)
        - Peripheral nerve injuries – related to diabetes or trauma

- Drug induced
    - Multiple drugs can interrupt nervous signals towards the bladder
    - Common culprits include:

- General Anaesthetic
- Antihistamines
- Anticholinergics
- Opiates
- NSAID's

Red Flags:

If urinary retention is accompanied with lower limb neurology, saddle anaesthesia or altered faecal continence consider cauda equina syndrome and arrange an urgent MRI of the spine. If not recognised and treated urgently neurological sequelae can be permanent.

The history:

- Preceding lower urinary tract symptoms or previous episodes of retention
- Is there an obvious recent precipitant: recent surgery/new drugs/constipation/known prostate disease/pelvic cancer
- Are there any systemic features of cancer?
- Are there any features of neurological disease or spinal injury?
    - Remember if appropriate to perform a full neurological exam

Investigations:

When examining the patient with urinary retention a rectal exam is essential. Not wanting to do it or not having done many before is **not a valid excuse**!

"If you don't put your finger in it, you'll put your foot in it!!"

Tips on an effective PR exam (figure 9):

- This is often unpleasant for patients, do everything you can to put them at ease
- Maintain patient modesty at all times
- Get a chaperone and where practical see if the patient would prefer a same-sex chaperone
- TELL THE PATIENT WHAT YOU ARE DOING/GOING TO DO
- Lie patient on left side and bring knees up to chest

- Examine the external anal aperture note any obvious haemorrhoids, masses or skin changes
- Using KY jelly, insert a finger into the anus, assess anal tone
- Note the presence of stool: Empty rectum or faecal loading
- Ensure to note the size and consistency of the prostate and ask if they have any discomfort. It is sensible to also assess the rectum as well.
- Remove the finger and look at the glove for the presence of blood
- Help the patient with hygiene and dressing, as needed

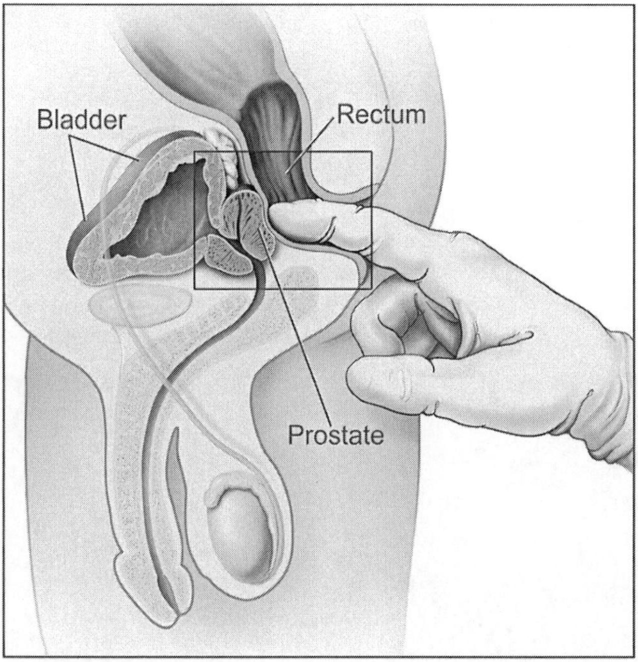

Figure 9. *Rectal Exam – note the position of the prostate* (Wikipedia 2008)

Blood tests:

- FBC – Infection/anaemia related to malignancy
- U&E – Obstructive uropathy
- CRP – infection

- Measuring prostate specific antigen (PSA) in acute retention is NOT recommended unless your rectal examination is indicative of prostate cancer. Retention and infection will artificially elevate the PSA and may condemn the patient to unnecessary investigations.

Imaging

- Bladder scan
    - An easy to use ward-level scan that can estimate the volume of urine in the bladder
    - Be aware of false positives from:
        - Ascites
        - Ovarian cysts

- Ultrasound Kidneys/ureters/bladder (figure 10)
    - Can estimate the size of the prostate & identify hydronephrosis
    - The adjacent ultrasound demonstrates hydronephrosis
    - Is not necessary in acute urinary retention unless you have a suspicion of high-pressure chronic retention or prostate cancer.

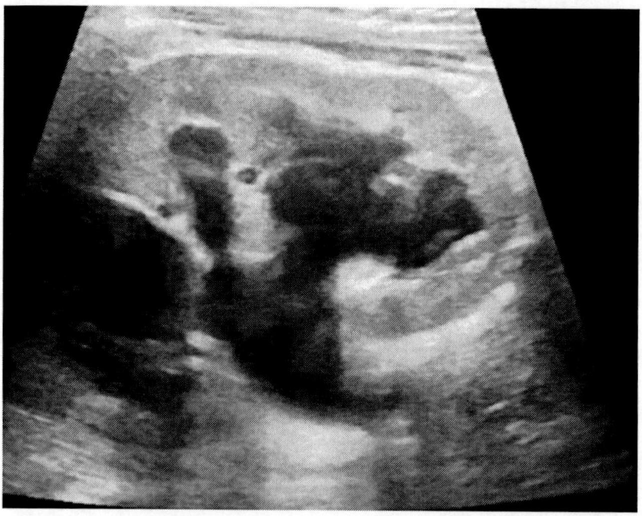

Figure 10. *Ultrasound showing evidence of hydronephrosis due to pelvicureteric obstruction (Wikipedia 2015)*

- CT or MRI spine may be required in specific situations as mentioned prior

Management

- As soon as retention has been confirmed: either with high clinical suspicion or bladder scan, the patient should be catheterised.

Tips for the difficult catheter:

- Put the patient at ease. Use a chaperone, use a quieter room and talk them through the process. This will make it easier.
- Get all the equipment ready on a sterile surface so there is no fumbling for kit during the activity.
- Use up to two syringes of local anaesthetic lubricant and give it time to work (beware – some patients are allergic to chlorhexidine, always check allergies with the patients before using this).
- In the male patient use gauze to hold the penis up vertically in the air.
- It may be easier to use a bigger catheter 16F + rather than smaller. 12Fr catheters are NOT recommended for male patients in retention.
- In the male if you encounter resistance, apply gentle steady pressure to pass through the obstruction. Do not repeatedly shove the catheter, this will cause a false passage. Although the prostate is blamed for many failed catheters, false passages are typically found in the bulbar urethra with the obstruction caused by a closed sphincter in tense, anxious patients.
- Advance the catheter to the hilt and **do not fill the balloon until urine starts to flow** and when it is filled used water rather than saline. There is potential for saline to crystallise in the balloon.
- Document the residual, whether the catheterisation was difficult and what colour urine comes out.
- If the patient has a foreskin – put it back where it was. Otherwise you will be managing the paraphimosis.
- In many cases the patient knows what works: ASK THEM.

Still can't catheterise?

- Curved tip catheter (figure 11)
    - Placing a catheter with a curved tip may allow the catheter to glide over an enlarged prostate.
    - The curve should point upward on insertion.

- Suprapubic catheterisation (SPC)
    - This should only be performed by an appropriately trained and competent person - your boss will be very happy to train you to do this procedure.
    - There is a risk of significant harm if not performed correctly
    - Before you do it discuss with a urologist first
    - Most guidelines highly recommend the use of ultrasound when siting a suprapubic catheter

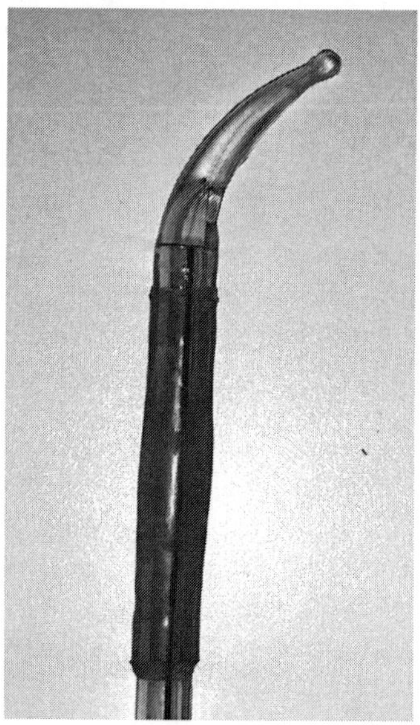

Figure 11. *Curved tip catheter.*

- Bladder aspiration
    - This is designed only to buy time for a definitive catheter plan

- Only when the bladder is palpable
- Use a green needle 2 finger breadths above the pubic symphysis and aspirate using the largest syringe possible until return is minimal

- When not to aspirate or place a suprapubic catheter:
  - Overlying cellulitis
  - History of previous bladder cancer
  - Presence of a femoral-femoral crossover graft
  - Pregnancy
  - Coagulopathic states
  - Impalpable bladder or not identified on ultrasound
  - Low abdominal wound
  - Inadequate training

Post catheterisation

- Record the residual volume, size of catheter, ease of insertion & colour of urine.
- Start tamsulosin (400mcg, oral, once daily) if thought to be prostate in nature. This increases the chance of a successful trial without catheter (TWOC).
- Organise further investigations as required related to the likely aetiology
- Treat other causes e.g. laxatives in constipation or finasteride in prostate disease
- Ensure there is a plan for follow up

The suprapubic catheter has fallen out

- Act quickly, before the tract closes
- Firstly, attempt to replace with the same size catheter
- If that fails, try dilating the tract with sequential Lofric catheters
- If the SPC still cannot be replaced, a urethral catheter should be placed until safe reinsertion of an SPC can be arranged

When to admit

This is contentious and resource dependent changing from different hospitals, however some situations include:

- Patients with renal dysfunction
- Patients with evidence of significant infection
- In cases related to haematuria
- Those who cannot manage their catheter
- Those with a residual volume >800mL after catheterisation
- Those with retention due to a critical aetiology requiring urgent management (i.e. spinal injury)

When to wake the boss:

- If no one can get a catheter in
- Remember this might not be the on call urologist - the surgical registrar or ED senior may be able to help

Further reading on urinary retention

- Teachmephysiology.com (Urinary)
    - Overview of the relevant physiology related to micturition
- NICE Clinical Knowledge Summary: LUTS in men
    - An overview of low urinary tract symptoms more appropriate for the outpatient and primary care setting
- Insertion of a suprapubic catheter (BAUS)
    - Patient leaflet discussing the benefits and risks of inserting a suprapubic catheter

Section 5: Haematuria

> *"Sorry to bother you doc. The patient has FRANK HAEMATURIA!"* – The medical nurse at 3am.

The questions the cross-cover doctor should ask at the time of referral?

- Has the patient had a bladder scan? Are they in retention?
- Are they in pain?
    - Painful haematuria is more related with inflammation & obstruction
- What do you mean by frank haematuria? It could be rose wine, Ribena, merlot, pure blood?
- Is the blood throughout the urinary stream?

  - Early only? - Think urethral
  - Continuous – Think throughout urinary tract
- Are there clots? What shape are they?
  - Clots indicate more extensive haematuria
  - If the clots are more string-like it could be associated with upper renal tract pathology
- Are they haemodynamically stable?
- Do they take anticoagulant medication? If so why? Is it safe to stop it or even reverse it if necessary?
- Are there any blood results yet?
- If it is indeed frank haematuria can someone place a 3-way catheter and start irrigation.

Definitions:

- Haematuria: Presence of blood in the urine
- Visible haematuria: Visible blood in the urine
- Non-visible haematuria (microscopic): Blood detected on urine dipstick

Figure 12. *Public patient information notice on urine colour.*
See colour centrefold for this image.

As figure 12 suggests a small volume of blood can have a drastic effect on the colour of the urine (Posilicious 2019)

Given the nature of this book the focus is on frank haematuria. It should be noted that non-visible haematuria may in some circumstances require further investigation.

Aetiology:

- Malignancy:
  - The positive predictive value for a male with visible haematuria in urological cancer is 20%. Therefore, visible haematuria is malignant until proven otherwise.
  - Bladder/ureteric/prostate/renal penile cancers can all present with haematuria and it might be the only symptom so it should be investigated as such.

- Infection:
    - Both lower and upper urinary tract infection have the potential to cause haematuria

- Stone disease:
    - Rarely ureteric stones can cause visible haematuria

- Prostate disease:
    - Hypervascular prostates in both benign and malignant prostate disease can cause haematuria

- Trauma:
    - Frank haematuria in trauma is commonly associated with renal injuries
    - All traumatic haematuria should be approached in regard to the ATLS algorithm first

- Intrinsic renal disease:
    - Should be thought of in younger patients
    - Can be associated nephritic syndrome and other intrinsic renal disease and if suspected a nephrology consult should be sought

- Haematological disease:
    - Myeloproliferative disorders and the use of anticoagulation may exacerbate haematuria, however it should not be primarily of thought of as aetiological.
    - These patients still require a full work up to investigate the haematuria

- Pseudo-haematuria (visible or microscopic haematuria without the presence of red blood cells in the urine):
    - Vaginal bleeding
    - Dyes in food & drugs e.g. beetroot & rifampacin
    - Myoglobinuria e.g. in rhabdomyolysis

- Iatrogenic:
    - Instrumentation
    - Urological surgery
    - Drug induced e.g. cyclophosphamide

Investigations

- Bedside:
    - Physical exam including rectal exam
    - Urinalysis
    - Bladder scan

- Blood tests:
    - FBC – Infection/anaemia related to malignancy
    - U&E – Obstructive uropathy
    - CRP – infection
    - Clotting – Rule out exacerbating coagulopathy
    - Measuring prostate specific antigen in an acute episode is NOT recommended. It can be twice the correct value up to a fortnight after the resolution of the retention episode
    - Group and Save/Cross matched blood – If the patient has bled to a point of significant anaemia or continues to bleed they may well require a blood transfusion

- Imaging:
    - USS KUB can identify some renal and bladder lesions and is a simple first line test
    - CT is used with non-contrast to identify stones and with contrast can identify or better categorise urothelial lesions.
    - MRI can better categorise certain urothelial lesions seen on other imaging modalities

- Specialist:
    - Outpatient flexible cystoscopy is mandatory in all patients with frank haematuria. There is no radiological test that supersedes this in identifying potential bladder tumours.

Acute management

- All patients should be resuscitated in regards to the ALS ABC algorithm
- Consider blood transfusion if the patient has lost a significant volume of blood or continues to bleed

- Consider reversing any anticoagulation. This requires a sensible risk assessment and should be based on local policy.
- Those with significant frank haematuria are at high risk of developing urinary retention secondary to a blood clot. The presenting feature may even be retention. If a patient presents with frank haematuria or clot retention, they require a 3-way catheter and frequent bladder washouts until the urine begins to clear.

The three-way catheter

- As the name suggests there are three channels (figure 13)
- One for urine to come out
- One to inflate the balloon
- The third allows for water to irrigate the bladder and prevent clot retention. It also allows for bladder washouts

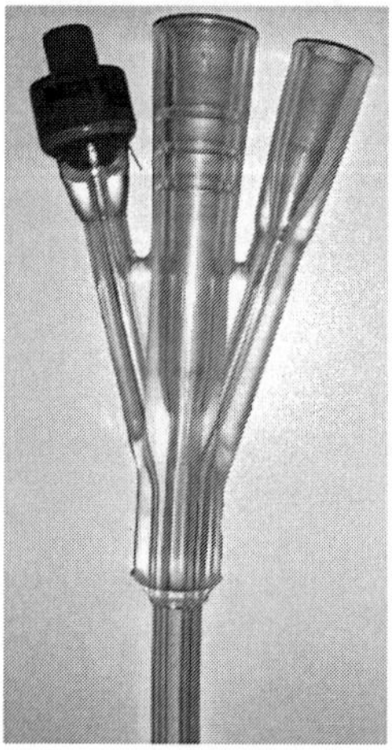

Figure 13. *Three-way catheter*

When the bleeding doesn't settle

- Tranexamic acid 1g TDS, an antifibrinolytic, may help settle the bleeding
- Gently pulling the catheter so it rests against the bladder neck may help aid in haemostasis. When the catheter is in this position it can be taped to the leg to keep it there

When to wake the boss

- Patients who are bleeding with haemodynamic compromise despite resuscitation
- Those with aetiologies that might require surgical intervention to stop the bleeding e.g. substantial trauma or significant post-operative bleeding

Further reading on haematuria

- NICE guideline suspected cancer: Recognition & referral
    - Further details on when and how to investigate suspected urological malignancies including those with visible & non-visible haematuria

Section 6: Foreskin emergencies

"Doctor, that patient you catheterised earlier, their penis is swollen and the foreskin doesn't look right" – The medical ward sister

Definitions

- Paraphimosis:
    - A condition in which the foreskin becomes retracted and fixed behind the glans penis (figure 14 – left image).
    - The resultant oedema can cause vascular compromise and if not corrected can result in ischaemic injury to glans if not corrected quickly.

- Phimosis:
    - Where the foreskin cannot be retracted behind the glans (figure 14 – right hand image)
    - Rarely a medical emergency
    - This will not be discussed here

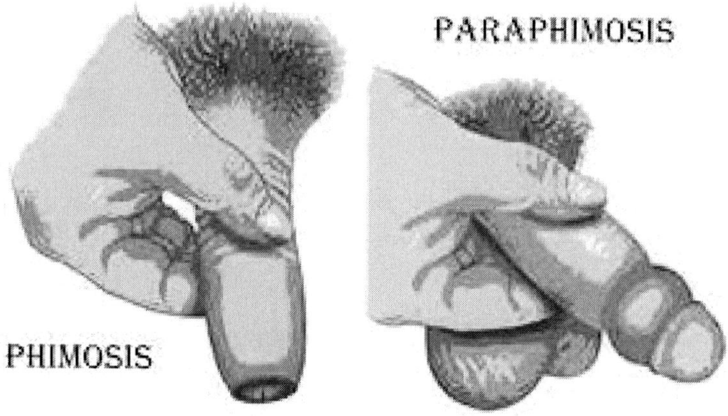

Figure 14. *Paraphimosis and phimosis* (cliniqonline 2019)

Red Flags:

In a patient with a paraphimosis with evidence of ischaemia, urgent reduction is required and possible surgery. If this is not possible by you get senior help fast.

Risk factors/Aetiology

- Iatrogenic e.g. failing to replace the foreskin after catheterisation
- Sexual activity
- Poor hygeine
- Balanitis
- Diabetes
- Penile piercing
- Pre-existing phimosis

Investigations

Diagnosis is clinical & further investigations are not necessary

Management

- Manual reduction:
    - Requires two people
        - One to do the procedure
        - The second to distract and talk to the patient
    - Tell the patient what you are doing! Do you best to get them relaxed
    - Lie the patient flat & give them a decent dose of analgesia prior to the procedure. They may even require a penile block.
    - Wrap one hand around the penis including the paraphimosis and apply steady and constant pressure.
    - Be patient! This may take 5 minutes; ask the distractor to monitor time.
    - After this time the swelling should have decreased
    - Then using both hands, press down on the glans with both thumbs and bring the phimosis ring above the glans.
    - If this doesn't work, try again.

- Multiple punctures
    - If manual reduction does not work, the Dundee method can be used
    - The odematous area is relatively insensate, but still may require a penile block prior to proceeding
    - Using one hand apply manual pressure as prior
    - Using a narrow brown needle and rapidly and repeatedly puncture the odematous area
    - This should remove enough fluid to proceed with manual reduction.

- Surgical reduction
    - If the above fails and usually under general anaesthetic, a dorsal slit may be required
    - This is followed by a later circumcision
    - It is performed in two stages to allow the oedema to settle and improve the rate of healing

Follow up
All patients should be discussed with urology for potential outpatient discussions regarding circumcision.

When to wake the boss?

- If you cannot reduce the foreskin despite initial steps
- If there is evidence of skin necrosis or vascular compromise

Section 7: Urological Trauma

The 8am trauma bleep: *"Trauma team to A&E resus. Ten minutes."*

Trauma golden rule: Follow ATLS principles!
Urologists rarely form part of the trauma team because they are usually not needed until a catheter is required, but the on-call surgical SHO and registrar are key components to this team. Remember the basics: Airway, Breathing & Circulation come first.

Most urological trauma is identified either at the Secondary Survey or more realistically on the pan-CT. In the event of significant urological injury e.g. renal trauma, you should have a low threshold to wake the boss, as this area is more specialist and delayed intervention may worsen prognosis.

Renal trauma

- Initial questions to ascertain:
    - Is the patient stable i.e. is it safe for imaging?
    - Full trauma picture i.e. other injuries - does this patient need to be transferred to a trauma centre?
    - Mechanism of injury: blunt vs penetrating, low vs high velocity force
    - Haematuria
    - Prior urological history

Incidence

- Occurs in as much as 10% of abdominal trauma
- Accounts for 3% of trauma admissions

Aetiology

Blunt abdominal/flank trauma is the most common mechanism in renal trauma. Falls, motor vehicle collisions & pedal bike accidents are associated most commonly.

- Blunt
  - The extent of deceleration in blunt trauma can predict the likelihood of the rarer, but more lethal renovascular injuries
- Penetrating injuries (Stab injuries, gunshot wounds)
- Iatrogenic (Renal biopsy)
- Spontaneous (In childbirth)

Presentation

- Traumatic setting
- Flank/abdominal pain
- Haematuria
- Rarely haemodynamic instability
- Co-existing ipsilateral rib fracture can increase the risk of renal injury threefold

Investigations (Renal specific, full trauma investigations & work up required)

- Bedside:
  - Urine dipstick
    - Visible and non-visible haematuria in the setting of trauma are good predictors of renal trauma.
    - However, the magnitude of haematuria does not correlate with the extent of the trauma and should not be used as a sole diagnostic tool.
- Imaging:
  - CT Urogram
    - The gold standard in genitourinary trauma imaging
    - An excretory phase is **ESSENTIAL** in suspected renal trauma as it is the only way to identify lacerations extending into the renal collecting system.

- Patient must be safe for the trip to the CT scanner
- Intravenous pyelography
    - Intravenous contrast followed by a delayed x ray KUB is useful in a life-saving operating table scenario, purely to confirm that a patient has the usual quota of kidneys before removing an injured one.

Staging renal trauma

AAST Grading	Injury description
1	• Contusion or non-expanding subcapsular haematoma
2	• Non-expanding peri-renal haematoma OR • Superficial (<1cm) laceration to the cortex with **NO** collecting system injury
3	• Superficial (>1cm) laceration to the cortex with **NO** collecting system injury
4	• Lacerations extending through the cortex & medulla with associated collecting duct injury OR • Renal artery or vein injury with contained haematoma
5	• Shattered kidney OR • Renal pedicle avulsion

Table 3. *American Association for the Surgery of Trauma grading for renal trauma*

Management

- Renal trauma is graded using the American Association for the Surgeons of Trauma (AAST) classification
- Grades 1-3 rarely need any intervention, only bedrest and perhaps an interval CT scan
- Grades 4-5 and penetrating injuries to the kidney may require operative management:
    - Arterial embolization

        - Surgical repair/emergency nephrectomy

Ureteric trauma

- Most commonly iatrogenic injury: gynaecological, colorectal and urological surgery
- Rare in blunt trauma, but when present is usually associated with polytrauma
- Features at presentation include:
    - Haematuria
    - Flank pain
    - Renal dysfunction
    - Sepsis from urinoma
- Gold standard for diagnosis is CT Urogram demonstrating extravasation of contrast outside of the urinary tract
- Management depends on the exact location and extent of the injury
- Minor injuries may be managed with ureteric stenting or nephrostomy whilst more severe injuries may require surgical reconstruction
- Many iatrogenic injuries are identified intra-operatively and a direct repair by a urologist can be performed

Bladder trauma

- Causes:
    - Non-iatrogenic:
        - Aetiology & management differs dependent on whether the rupture is intra or extraperitoneal
            - Intraperitoneal: Results from sudden increased pressure of a full bladder due to acute blunt force
            - Extraperitoneal: Almost always associated with pelvic fractures
    - Iatrogenic:
        - Commonly injured during obstetric, gynaecological & urological procedures
- Presentation:
    - Visible haematuria
    - Abdominal pain & distension
    - Sepsis
    - Reduced urine output

- CT with contrast is the most commonly used diagnostic modality
- Management:
    - Intraperitoneal bladder ruptures are more likely to lead to peritonitis & sepsis and should be repaired – it is usually done via a laparotomy
    - Extraperitoneal bladder ruptures are more likely to be managed conservatively with urinary catheterisation, IV antibiotics and suitable follow up with a cystogram.

Urethral Trauma

- Most commonly iatrogenic and related to invasive procedures such as: catheterisation, transurethral surgery as well as surgical and oncological treatment for urological malignancies
- Non-iatrogenic causes include: motor vehicle accidents, straddle injuries, penile fractures, pelvic fractures and rarely penetrating injuries.
- Presentation:
    - Blood at urethral meatus
    - Inability to void with a palpable bladder
    - Haematuria
    - Inability to pass urethral catheter
    - High-riding/impalpable prostate on trauma DRE
- Diagnosis is based on retrograde urethrography with cystoscopy used to assess the degree of injury further.
- Treatment:
    - Catheterisation
        - One attempt at urethral catheterisation by an experienced individual is reasonable
        - Flexible cystoscopic guided catheterisation may be possible
        - Suprapubic catheterisation under ultrasound guidance is appropriate
    - Definitive treatment is dependent on the mechanism, area of the urethra injured & co-existing injuries.

Penile & Scrotal trauma

- Penile fractures
    - Rupture of the tunica albuginea most commonly related to blunt trauma to the erect penis

- May be associated with urethral injury
- Most commonly related to sexual intercourse, masturbation & cultural practices of penile bending
- Presentation
    - Swelling & painful penis (eggplant penis)
    - Immediate loss of erection (detumescence)
    - Cracking noise
- Diagnosis
    - Clinical
    - Ultrasound
    - 10% penile fractures have a concurrent urethral injury: cystoscopy or retrograde urethrography can diagnose this
- Surgical repair with closure of the tunica albuginea should be undertaken in all cases to prevent deformity and maintain erectile function – you will need the boss for this.

- Scrotal trauma
    - Haematocele
        - Collection of blood in the scrotal sac
        - Large haematoceles require surgical exploration
    - Testicular rupture
        - Related to high energy blunt trauma
        - On examination the affected hemiscrotum is tender and bruised with the testicle being difficult to palpate
        - Ultrasound can aid diagnosis
        - Testicular ruptures should be surgically repaired

Further reading on haematuria

- European Associations of Urology: Urological Trauma:
    - Comprehensive review of urological trauma

Section 9: Priapism

The emergency department whiteboard shows a 50-year-old gentleman with "personal problems". The triage nurse says: "It isn't going down doc".

Definitions:

- A persistent erection prolonged over four hours in the absence of sexual desire
- Incidence of 2.9/100,000 in males over 40
- Many differing and unexpected aetiologies

The questions the cross-cover doctor should ask at the time of referral?

- Duration of erection
- Pain?
- First episode?
- Urological history?
- Trauma history?
- Co-existing medical problems: malignancy, haematological disease & drugs

Types of priapism & differing presentations:

- Low flow priapism (Ischaemic):
  - Secondary to inadequate venous & lymphatic drainage from the corpus cavernosae
  - Presentation:
    - Persistent and painful
    - Unrelated to sexual stimulus
  - Low flow (Ischaemic) priapism lasting more than 4 hours is an emergency.

- High flow priapism:
  - Secondary to unregulated increased arterial flow
  - Rarer than low flow
  - Presentation:
    - Painless
    - Usually trauma related e.g. saddle injuries
    - May present recurrently
    - Penis not fully rigid

These can be distinguished based on aspiration results of corporal blood

Aetiology:

- Medication
  - Erectile dysfunction medication
  - Cocaine
  - Antipsychotics/Antihypertensives/Antidepressants

- Haematological
  - Hypercoagulable states seen in sickle cell, leukaemia or thrombophilia may lead to priapism

- Neurological
  - Related to certain spinal conditions such as spinal shock, cauda equina, MS or certain spinal cord tumours

- Trauma
  - More commonly in high flow priapism – trauma to the genitalia or perineum can result in a fistula leading to priapism.

Investigations & Initial Management

The mainstay of treatment is to preserve erectile function, manage pain & prevent tissue loss

- 'ABC' approach:
  - The priapism could be the distracting aspect of the presentation

- Analgesia:
  - The patient will thank you and make thorough assessment much easier

- Ice packs:
  - May help aid detumescence in the initial setting

- Bloods:
  - A full blood count and differential may point towards the aetiology e.g. leukaemia or sickle cell causing anaemia
  - Corpus cavernosum blood sampling

        - Sampling the blood from the corpus cavernosum can distinguish between high & low flow priapism with high flow samples representing those similar to those found in arterial blood.
        - This is discussed further in the management section

- Imaging:
    - Ultrasound with duplex
    - Penile arteriography

When to wake the boss:

- Delays or improper treatment may be result in permanent loss of erection; if you are unfamiliar with its management you should discuss it with a urologist even if this means phoning a tertiary centre.

Definitive Management

Low flow & High flow priapism are managed differently:

- Low flow priapism
    - Cavernosal aspiration +/- irrigation
    - Performed under a penile block
    - Insert a butterfly needle in to the cavernosum and aspirate blood (this can be tested simultaneously to aid diagnosis) at either the 2 or 10 o'clock position. This avoids the urethra and major vessels.
    - The corpus cavernosum can be simultaneously irrigated with a sympathomimetic such as phenylephrine – you may have to get this from obstetrics, ICU or the pharmacy
    - Due to its cardiac effects the use of such drugs should be done with cardiac monitoring
    - This can be repeated as required.
    - Surgical treatments:
        - If aspiration and irrigation fails or if the priapism has lasted longer than 48 hours at presentation, surgical drainage may be required
        - Under a general anaesthetic there are three commonly used methods of shunting blood from the corpus cavernosum

- High flow priapism
    - Initial observation
    - Pressure on the perineum may aid resolution
    - In patients seeking treatment arteriography and embolization or surgery can be curative

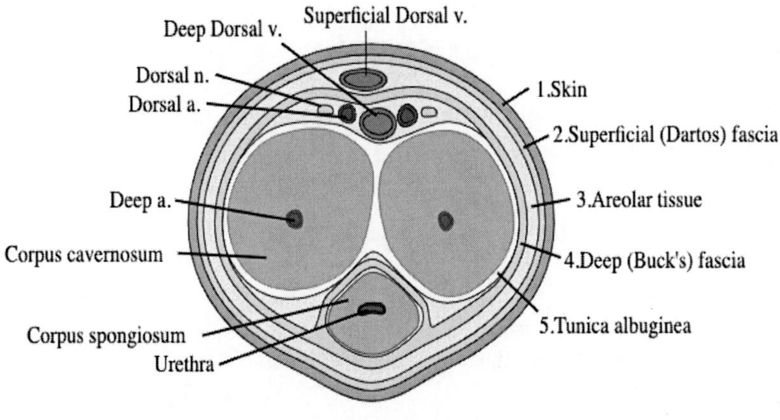

Figure 15. *Cross-section of the penis. When aspirating a priapism, the needle should enter at the 2 & 10 o'clock position avoiding the vasculature & urethra.* (Wikipedia 2013)

Further reading on priapism

- Cherian J, Rao AR, Thwaini A, Kapasi F, Shergill IS, Samman R. Medical and surgical management of priapism. Postgraduate Medical Journal. 2006 Feb 1;82(964):89-94. This gives a detailed explanation of the surgical options in priapism with detailed diagrams

Section 10: The Spectrum of Infection

Ward nurse at 3am: *"Hi Doctor, we put a catheter in the 90-year-old after her laparotomy. She's well but her urine dipstick is positive for everything. Would you prescribe some antibiotics for her UTI?"*

Background

Most straightforward urinary tract infections do not require hospital admission, but they particularly do not need a urological admission. Some general advice concerning urinary tract infection is included below, as well as the management of more significant infections.

Simple Lower Urinary Tract Infection

The urinalysis can be a useful tool in management of those with a *symptomatic* urinary tract infection.

Typical urinary symptoms include:

- Dysuria,
- A short-history of frequency and urgency
- Malodourous urine
- Haematuria and it can be quite significant.
- Fever and rigors

Patients with clear history of infection should have a urine MC&S sent and appropriate antibiotics initiated.

A positive dipstick: Leucocytes AND nitrites AND symptomatic infection.

- Blood and protein is not a positive dipstick
- Leucocytes in isolation is not a positive dipstick
- Ketones mean the patient is not eating adequately
- A high specific gravity means the patient is dehydrated
- Glucose means they are either diabetic or should be investigated for it!
- Protein can indicate renovascular disease

Beware asymptomatic bacteriuria

- Very common in >65yrs females
- Often over-treated
- If they don't describe symptoms of infection, they do NOT need antibiotics

Complicated Lower Urinary Tract Infection

- Bladder infection (cystitis) in Men
    - UTI in men is uncommon and should be appropriately investigated to identify a potential underlying cause such as bladder stones and bladder outflow obstruction
    - They may require an ultrasound of the urinary tract, a flexible cystoscopy or flow-rate assessment.
- Recurrent UTI in Women
    - Doesn't need a hospital admission but should be followed up in urology outpatients
    - Needs a careful history by a urologist and may need a flexible cystoscopy

- Epididymo-orchitis
    - Typically presents with a short history of a red, hot and swollen hemi-scrotum – patients are exquisitely tender, and the testicle may be very hard on examination
    - Young men should be treated with a low index of suspicion for sexually transmitted infections (STIs) and should be counselled to attend a sexual health clinic.
    - Older men typically develop this infection related to a UTI and should be investigated as above
    - Each hospital will have its own recommended antibiotics, most units utilise fluoroquinolones such as ciprofloxacin
    - An ultra-sounds scan of the testes will confirm a diagnosis but is not essential unless you suspect an abscess

- Prostatitis
    - Divided into two main groups: Acute bacterial and chronic prostatitis (chronic pelvic pain syndrome)
    - Acute bacterial infections are associated with pelvic, perineal and genital pain, fever and rigors and often dysuria.
    - A rectal examination is essential and may identify a boggy and tender prostate
    - This is again treated with a long course (2-6/52) of fluoroquinolones, NSAIDS and occasionally an alpha-blocker.
    - Do NOT send a PSA during acute infection

Upper urinary tract infection (pyelonephritis)

This group is divided into simple and complicated. Pyelonephritis is characterised by fever and rigors, loin pain and night sweats; patients may describe recent or co-existing lower urinary tract symptoms. Patients with minor UTIs will often described infections 'going to their kidneys'. True pyelonephritis patients can often be frighteningly unwell with significant sepsis signs such as hypotension and persistent pyrexia. Most will respond very well to IV fluid resuscitation and IV antibiotics.

Simple pyelonephritis

This is typically found in young females and is usually managed with an USS Kidneys and IV antibiotics by our physician colleagues. A urology admission is not necessary.

Complex pyelonephritis

- Beware the missed septic obstructing stone
- Renal abscess
- Immunocompromised patients
- Pyelonephritis in a man – myth or reality?

Fournier's gangrene

This is the rarest but arguably the most significant urological emergency. This is necrotising fasciitis of the genitals and perineum and early recognition is paramount to a patient surviving this diagnosis. It is a fulminant, rapidly progressing infection that spreads through tissue planes often affecting the immunosuppressed, alcoholic and poorly nourished, the diabetic and those with complex co-morbidities.

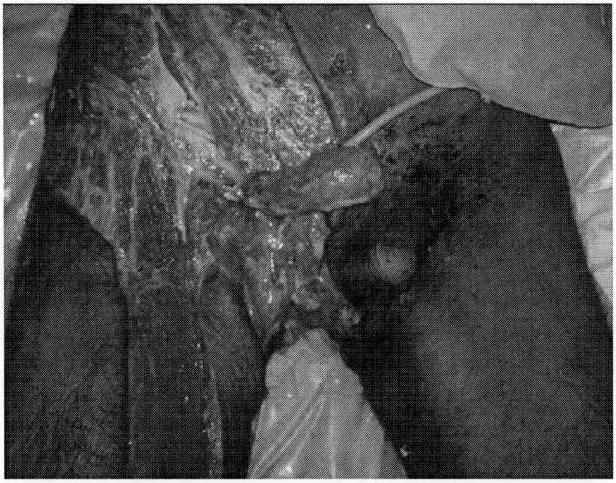

Figure 16. *A patient after extensive debridement for Fournier's gangrene. Note the urethral catheter in situ and colostomy bag (Wikipedia 2009)*

Symptoms/Signs

These are all red flags in any soft tissue examination

- Erythema of scrotal skin
- Sudden swelling/pain
- Rapidly progressing cellulitis – this infection will spread as you look at it
- Crepitus
- Necrotic patches are a late sign (Figure 17)

Management

- Resuscitation and quickly
- Broad-spectrum antibiotics – you will need to call the microbiologist as soon as possible
- Phone the boss immediately! Even in cases where you are not 100% sure, you should discuss with a senior and escalate
- Get the anaesthetist/ICU involved – patients will need inotropes and usually ICU for post-op pain management
- Get the patient to the emergency theatre as quick as you can – yes you can stop elective lists, yes you can bump that 'hot gallbladder'

and the laparotomy for small bowel obstruction. If this is not managed appropriately the patient will die.

- The only way to cure this is to debride the affected skin until it's gone; this process is tremendously disfiguring for patients but our plastic surgery colleagues will do amazing work further down the line.
- These patients should be debrided immediately and they should not be transferred for debridement.

References

American Association for the Surgery of Trauma, "Renal Trauma". Accessed 01/04/2019 http://www.aast.org/Library/TraumaTools/InjuryScoringScales.aspx#kidney

Bestpractice.bmj.com, "Testicular torsion - Symptoms, diagnosis and treatment". Accessed 27/02/2019. Available at: https://bestpractice.bmj.com/topics/en-gb/506

Bestpractice.bmj.com. "Priapism - Symptoms, diagnosis and treatment". Accessed 27/02/2019. Available at https://bestpractice.bmj.com/topics/en-gb/505

British Association for Urological Surgeons (BAUS). "Patient leaflets, Testicular Torsion". Accessed 27/02/2019. Available at: https://www.baus.org.uk/userfiles/pages/files/Patients/Leaflets/Torsion%20of%20testis.pdfBaus.org.uk

British Association Of Urological Surgeons (BAUS), "Insertion of a Suprapubic Catheter". Accessed 27/02/2019. Available at: https://www.baus.org.uk/_userfiles/pages/files/Patients/Leaflets/Suprapubic.pdf

British Association of Urological Surgeons, "Patient Leaflets – Percutaneous Nephrostomy". Accessed 27/02/2019. Available at: https://www.baus.org.uk/_userfiles/pages/files/Patients/Leaflets/Percutaneous%20nephrostomy.pdf

Campbell, Meredith F et al. 2016. *Campbell-Walsh urology*. Philadelphia: Elsevier.

Cherian, J. 2006. "Medical and surgical management of priapism". *Postgraduate Medical Journal* 82 (964): 89-94. BMJ. doi:10.1136/pgmj.2005.037291.

CliniQ, "Phimosis & Paraphimosis". Accessed 01/04/2019 https://cliniqonline.wordpress.com/2018/04/25/phimosis-and-paraphimosis/

Emedicine.medscape.com, "Urinary Obstruction: Practice Essentials, Background & Pathophysiology". Accessed 27/02/2019. Available at: https://emedicine.medscape.com/article/778456-overview

Emedicine.medscape.com. "Priapism: Practice Essentials, Background, Pathophysiology". Accessed 27/02/2019. Available at: https://emedicine.medscape.com/article/437237-overview

Ezez. 2018. *Advanced trauma life support*. Chicago, IL: American College of Surgeons

Flickr, "Take the urine colour test". Accessed 01/04/2019 https://www.flickr.com/photos/derekmorrison/4792771887

Kaisary, Amir V et al. 2016. *Lecture notes*. Chichester, West Sussex: John Wiley & Sons Inc.

Learning.bmj.com, "Surgical skills - exploration of scrotum for testicular torsion". Accessed 27/02/2019. Available at: https://learning.bmj.com/learning/module-intro/scrotum-testicular-torsion.html?locale=en_GB&moduleId=10033430

Mayo Clinic, "Testicular torsion - Symptoms and causes". Accessed 27/02/2019. Available at: https://www.mayoclinic.org/diseases-conditions/testicular-torsion/symptoms-causes/syc-20378270

Mokhmalji, Hassan et al. 2001. "Percutaneous nephrostomy versus ureteral stents for diversion of hydronephrosis caused by stones: A prospective, randomised clinical trial.". *The Journal of Urology*: 1088-1092. Ovid Technologies (Wolters Kluwer Health). doi:10.1097/00005392-200104000-00007

National Cancer Institute, "Digital Rectal Exam". Accessed 01/04/2019 https://visualsonline.cancer.gov/details.cfm?imageid=4351

NHS UK, "Rectal Examination". Accessed 27/02/2019. Available at: https://www.nhs.uk/conditions/rectal-examination/

NICE: Clinical Knowledge Summary. "Lower Urinary Tract Symptoms in Men". Accessed 27/02/2019. Available at https://cks.nice.org.uk/luts-in-men#!backgroundsub:1

NICE: Clinical Knowledge Summary. "Urological cancers - recognition and referral". Accessed 27 Feb. 2019. Available at: https://cks.nice.org.uk/urological-cancers-recognition-and-referral#!scenario

NICE. "Lower Urinary Tract Infection Guideline". Accessed 27/02/2019. Available at: https://www.guidelines.co.uk/urology/nice-lower-urinary-tract-infection-guideline/454434.article

Pearle, Margaret. et al. 1998. "Optimal method of urgent decompression of the collecting system for obstruction and infection due to ureteral calculi". *The Journal of Urology*: 1260-1264. Ovid Technologies (Wolters Kluwer Health). doi:10.1097/00005392-199810000-00013.

Pickard, Robert et al. 2015. "Medical expulsive therapy in adults with ureteric colic: a multicentre, randomised, placebo-controlled trial". *The Lancet* 386 (9991): 341-349. Elsevier BV. doi:10.1016/s0140-6736 (15)60933-3

Pixabay, "Testicles". Accessed 01/04/2019. (public domain) https://pixabay.com/photos/testicles-testicular-cancer-penis-2790218/

Public domain Pictures, "Back Pain". Accessed 01/04/2019(public domain). https://www.publicdomainpictures.net/en/view-image.php?image=237870&picture=back-pain

Sheth, K., Keays, M., Grimsby, G., Granberg, C., Menon, V., DaJusta, D., Ostrov, L., Hill, M., Sanchez, E., Kuppermann, D., Harrison, C., Jacobs, M., Huang, R., Burgu, B., Hennes, H., Schlomer, B. and Baker, L (2016). "Diagnosing Testicular Torsion before Urological Consultation and Imaging: Validation of the TWIST Score". Journal of Urology, 195(6), pp.1870-1876.

TeachMePhysiology, "Micturition". Accessed 27/02/2019. Available at http://teachmephysiology.com/urinary-system/micturition/

Türk, Christian et al. 2016. "EAU Guidelines on Interventional Treatment for Urolithiasis". *European Urology* 69 (3): 475-482. Elsevier BV. doi:10.1016/j.eururo.2015.07.041.

UROWEB. "Urological Trauma". Accessed 27/02/2019. Available at: https://uroweb.org/guideline/urological-trauma

Wikimedia Commons, "Fournier Gangrene", Accessed 01/04/2019 https://commons.wikimedia.org/wiki/File:Fournier_gangrene_01.jpg

Wikimedia Commons, "Abdominal film with urethral stent", Accessed 01/04/2019 https://commons.wikimedia.org/wiki/File:Abdominal_Xray_with_uretal_stent.jpg

Wikimedia Commons, "KUB stone", Accessed 01/04/2019 https://commons.wikimedia.org/wiki/File:KUB_stone.jpg

Wikimedia Commons, "Nephrostomy", Accessed 01/04/2019 https://commons.wikimedia.org/wiki/Category:Nephrostomy

Wikimedia Commons, "Penis Cross Section", Accessed 01/04/2019 https://commons.wikimedia.org/wiki/File:Penis_cross_section.svg

Wikipedia. "Paraphimosis". Accessed 27/02/2019. Available at: https://en.wikipedia.org/wiki/Paraphimosis

Wikipedia. "Phimosis". Accessed 27/02/2019. Available at: https://en.wikipedia.org/wiki/Phimosis

Wikimedia Commons, "Testicular Torsion". Accessed 01/04/2019. https://commons.wikimedia.org/wiki/File:Hodendrehung_Post-OP.jpg

Wikimedia Commons, "Ultrasonography with hydronephrosis". Accessed 01/04/2019. https://commons.wikimedia.org/wiki/File:Ultrasonography_of_hydronephrosis_with_dilated_anechoic_pelvis_and_calyces,_along_with_cortical_atrophy_-_measurement.jpg

Wikimedia Commons, "Urinary Retention", Accessed 01/04/2019 https://commons.wikimedia.org/wiki/File:Urinary_retention.jpg

Ye, Zhangqun et al. 2010. "A multicentre, prospective, randomized trial: comparative efficacy of tamsulosin and nifedipine in medical expulsive therapy for distal ureteric stones with renal colic". *BJU International* 108 (2): 276-279. Wiley. doi:10.1111/j.1464-410x.2010.09801.x.

CHAPTER 9

VASCULAR SURGERY

TOM PAMPIGLIONE

Abstract
Section 1 – Vascular Networks
Section 2 – Assessment of vascular patients
The vascular patient
History
Vascular examination
Arterial
Venous
Special Tests
ABPI
Section 3 – Peripheral arterial disease
Intermittent claudication
Critical limb ischaemia
Acute limb ischaemia
Section 4 – Aortic disease
Ruptured Abdominal Aortic Aneurysm
Aortic Dissection
Aortic Dissection
Section 5 – Ulcers
Venous ulcers
Arterial ulcers
Neuropathic ulcers
Necrotic Toes
Diabetic Foot

Abstract

Vascular emergencies can be life or limb threatening. The way in which they present can be much more 'time critical' compared with other surgical specialties. Due to the changing nature of surgical training, hospitals with vascular units are developing specific on call rotas. However, in district general hospitals, there will still be times where emergencies are managed by doctors with little day to day vascular experience. It is vital that those covering this speciality are able to identify key warning signs, triage patients appropriately and perform an effective vascular examination.

This chapter covers key vascular emergencies and common non-emergency referrals including rupture of abdominal aortic aneurysm, critical limb ischaemia and ulcers. Often these patients will require emergency imaging, Senior surgical involvement and operative intervention. Vascular surgery registrars commonly provide non-resident cover. The role of the Senior House Officer is vital to coordinate these events and to facilitate the timely management of these patients.

Finally, we offer some tricks and tips for performing vascular examinations, including taking ankle-brachial pressure index measurements.

Section 1: Vascular Networks

Although currently there is no national vascular network, as in trauma, many areas have local agreements. These tend to operate in 2 main ways. Firstly, multiple large hospitals within a region may have a local rota as to where emergency vascular cases will be admitted. This allows there to be regional 24/7 coverage from senior surgeons who are regularly performing major arterial surgery.

Alternatively, they may operate in a "hub and spoke" model, where smaller vascular units may be linked with tertiary vascular centres. Typically, this happens between district general hospitals and teaching hospitals. Often non-urgent cases can be admitted overnight at the local hospital to be assessed in the morning, whereas vascular emergencies will be transferred directly to the tertiary centre. This ensures that major arterial surgery occurs in centres that regularly perform emergencies. This is not just due to the experience of the surgeons but also anaesthetists who are familiar with vascular surgery and intensive care unit availability. The tertiary hospital vascular surgery consultants may perform outreach clinics and elective surgery, usually venous, in the smaller centres.

It is essential that when starting any new post, you familiarise yourself with the local protocols and procedures. You may be covering patients at either end of these arrangements. You must know how and when to arrange a transfer to a receiving hospital. You may also be in a position where you have to decide which patients are to be transferred over to you. Reviewing local guidelines will ensure transfers are not only urgent but also appropriate. Tertiary centres cannot accept all referrals as usually regional admissions will be for many specialties. This would create a strain on resources. You may be the gatekeeper.

Section 2: Assessment of vascular patients

The 'vascular patient'

Problems that require input from a vascular surgeon are typically the sequelae of other medical comorbidities. These are typically cardiovascular in origin but can also commonly involve endocrine, connective tissue disease and other genetic conditions. When treating an unwell patient, it is important to appreciate the effect that their other medical conditions will have on their current presentation. Therefore, it is essential that care and attention is given to the whole picture.

History

In vascular surgery patients often present with acute or chronic pain. It is important to ascertain the nature of the pain. Vascular surgery patients, particularly those with arterial disease, often describe a characteristic pattern of pain (Table 1).

Where is the pain?	Common sites include calves, buttocks, feet or abdomen
When did the pain start?	Has this been going on for many months, is it progressing?

What is the character of the pain?	Patients often describe constant cramping or heavy pains rather than sharp, stabbing, intermittent pains.
Does the patient have pain in front of you now?	Do they have rest pain?
If the pain is intermittent, what are the triggers?	How long after walking does the pain come on, is it always a similar amount of time?
If exertional, how long before pain starts and is it relieved be cessation of activity	Does resting ease the pain.

Table 1. Pain questions

Past medical history:

- Has the patient had any previous surgery or input from vascular surgery before?
- It is essential to ascertain if a patient has had previous vascular intervention as this may be pertinent to their presentation.
- Have they had previous endovascular intervention or bypass procedures? Grafts or stents may become occluded
- Are they being monitored or managed conservatively for a pre-existing condition such as an abdominal aortic aneurysm or intermittent claudication
- Do they have risk factors for cardiovascular disease?
- Do they suffer from hypertension, diabetes, dyslipidaemia, obesity or chronic kidney disease?
- Male sex and increasing age are also risk factors for atherosclerosis
- Do they smoke?
- Do they have a strong family history?
- Did a 1st degree relative have a myocardial infarction, particularly at a young age?
- What medications do they take?
- Do they take anything which could predispose them to either bleeding or thrombosis?

Vascular examination

Vascular examinations are often targeted to either the arterial or venous system. However, it is important have an appreciation for both when making your assessment as patients will often have mixed disease.

> Top Tip!
> It can often be difficult and time consuming to gain an adequate exposure. It is often tempting to examine patients in their clothes or in a sub optimal position. However, you can often be caught out by missing previous surgery, wounds or other signs that the patient may have forgotten about!

Position and inspection:
As a minimum, patients should be exposed in such a way that all main pulses are accessible and both legs, including feet, are fully visible. They should be on an examination couch at a 45-degree angle.

Inspect around the patient's bedside

- Are there any walking aids?
- Check footwear, are they wearing a supportive boot?
- Any signs of smoking?
- Is their breathing restricted, do they look comfortable?
- Check for surgical scars
- Common relevant scars include:
- Midline sternotomy
- Laparotomy
- Vein harvest sites in legs
- Scars from previous groin explorations
- Amputations

Now inspect more closely:

Face

- Check for pallor and central cyanosis
- Xantholasma
- Corneal arcus
- Poor dental hygiene in smoking

Lower limb

- Arterial disease:
    - Hypotrophic changes
    - Thin skin
    - Hair loss
    - Muscle Wasting
    - Arterial ulcer
        - Punched out
        - Deep
        - Painful
        - Necrotic or sloughy top layer

- Venous disease:
    - Varicose veins
    - Venous eczema
    - Haemosiderin deposition
    - Lipodermatosclerosis
    - Inverted "champagne bottle appearance"
    - Ulceration

- Ischaemic toes:
    - Wet or dry gangrene
    - Check the level of demarcation
    - Is there an ulcer tracking to an interphalangeal joint – indicative of osteomyelitis
    - Check between the toes and on the plantar surface of the foot for ulcers and discolouration

- Open wounds: Check under the heels for broken skin or pressure necrosis
- Charcot foot: Deformity of the foot, secondary to peripheral neuropathy in diabetes. Subluxation and disclocation of the fore and midfoot leads to flattening, inversion and a "floppy" foot.

Arterial Examination

Palpation:

- Pulse
- Check the right radial pulse
- Check for rate, rhythm and character

- Capillary refill time: At hand, Centrally (sternum), Hallux
    - < 3 seconds in normal

- Temperature
    - Check at hand and feet
    - Is it symmetrical between limbs?
    - Cool in arterial disease - move proximally, where does it begin to warm?

- After this, it is acceptable to simply check for the presence of a pulse (Table 2)

Artery	Location
Radial	Proximal to the wrist joint in the groove lateral to the flexor tendons
Ulnar	Proximal to the wrist joint in the groove medial to the flexor tendons
Brachial	Anterior aspect of the elbow, medial to the biceps tendon
Carotid	Middle third of anterior border of sternocleidomastoid
Superficial temporal	Anterior to the tragus of the ear, superior to the zygomatic arch
Femoral	Mid inguinal point. Midway between a line drawn from the anterior superior iliac spine to the pubic symphysis
Popliteal	Place both hands around the knee from anteriorly. Rest your thumbs on the tibial tuberosity and fingers in the popliteal fossa. Lift your fingers to flex the knee slightly.
Posterior Tibial	In the groove approximately 2cm posterior and 2cm inferior to the medial malleolus
Dorsalis Paedis	Between the tendons of extensor hallucis longus and extensor digitorum longus of the second toe

Table 2. Pulse Anatomy

Top Tip! - Popliteal Pulse
This can be difficult to palpate. It is best felt at the inferior edge of the popliteal fossa. Both too much, and not enough pressure, will make it tricky to feel the pulse. If you are unable to find it, vary the knee flexion. If it extremely easy to palpate, then it may be aneurysmal.

- Examine for an abdominal aortic aneurysm
    - Palpate with 2 hands in the midline, between the xiphisternum and umbilicus
    - Check for a mass which is both pulsatile *and* expansile

Auscultation:
Auscultate for carotid bruits - this can indicate carotid stenosis

Lower limb:

- Examine sensation
    - Start distally at toes
    - Check for paraesthesia
    - Is it in a glove and stocking distribution, or dermatomal?

- Check movement
- Gross movement of toes is lost in acute limb ischaemia

Venous examination

Inspection forms the mainstay of a venous examination. It is essential to gain adequate exposure of the legs and feet.

Varicose veins are dilated tortuous veins that run across a territory. They can be associated with thrombophlebitis. This is where the vein may be inflamed or tender to touch.

- Long saphenous vein: this runs medially from the saphenofemoral junction in the groin to the anterior border of the medial malleolus

- Short saphenous vein: this originates posteriorly to the lateral malleolus, runs along the lateral border of the calf where it drains into the popliteal vein at the popliteal fossa

Venous signs or ulcers can be described as "in the territory" of the long or short saphenous vein depending on their location

Palpate for:

- Pitting oedema
- Distribution – what is the anatomical location or territory. E.g. mid-thigh or long saphenous vein?
- Thrombophlebitis
- Peripheral pulses (to ensure that it is not mixed arterio-venous disease)
- If compression bandaging is required (in this case perform Ankle Brachial Pressure Index [ABPI])

Special Tests:

Arterial

Buerger's test - tests for lower limb arterial insufficiency:

- With the patient supine, raise both feet to 45 degrees
- Hold the position for 2 minutes
- Look for:
    - Pallor of feet
    - Measure the angle at which pallor starts
- After 2 minutes sit the patient up, swing them 90 degrees and hang their feet over the side of the bed
- Look for:
    - Reactive hyperaemia - erythema of the feet when blood flow is restored, indicates arterial disease

Venous

Historically an examination called a tourniquet test has been described to ascertain the level of venous incompetence. However, in modern surgical practice venous duplex ultrasonography forms the gold standard for assessing venous reflux. Therefore, there is no longer a requirement to perform a tourniquet test to assess the level at which reflux originates. This is both an inaccurate test and has little impact on the management. A tap test is a crude measure that may be performed. However, this is only likely to be positive in patients where the varicosities are already obvious.

Tap test:
Lightly place your finger distally on the vein being assessed. Now tap on the vein around 15cm more proximally. A palpable fluid thrill at the distal finger indicates valvular incompetence.

Ankle Brachial Pressure Index

The ABPI is a clinical measurement which is used, in conjunction with clinical examination, to assess the flow of arterial blood to the lower limbs. It is derived by calculating the ratio between the systolic blood pressures of the brachial and the posterior tibial or dorsalis paedis arteries. The pressure at the brachial artery is an estimate of the central systolic pressure. This measurement estimates a reduction in arterial flow to the foot that can occur with atherosclerosis. This is of particular importance when applying pressure bandaging to treat venous ulcers, as it can instigate ischaemia of the foot in patients with mixed arterial/venous disease. A doppler ultrasound probe is used for accuracy.

Equipment required:
Manual Sphygmomanometer (BP cuff), hand held doppler probe, ultrasound gel (standard lubrication jelly is sufficient)

How to perform an ABPI:

- The patient must be placed supine. Having the patient reclined, or sat up, will overestimate the result.
- Place the sphygmomanometer cuff on the upper arm, as for a standard blood pressure reading.
- Place the doppler probe over the brachial artery so the signal may be heard
- Slowly inflate the cuff until the doppler signal is lost, continue for a further 20 mmHg beyond this point.
- Now carefully deflate the cuff. The point at which your doppler signal becomes audible again is your systolic blood pressure
- Repeat this procedure on the contralateral arm. The highest value should be included in the ratio
- Place the sphygmomanometer cuff over the mid-calf of the leg you are assessing.
- Now place the doppler probe over the dorsalis-paedis artery
- Inflate the cuff and measure the systolic pressure as per the brachial artery

- Move the doppler probe to the posterior tibial artery
- Take the highest systolic pressure from the foot and include this in the ratio
- Repeat for the contralateral lower limb if required

Calculation of ABPI and interpretation of results (Table 3):

- The ABPI is calculated by dividing the higher pressure of either foot pulses, on the limb being assessed, with the highest brachial pressure.
- For example, the dorsalis paedis and posterior tibial the measurements were 104 and 116 respectively. The highest brachial pressure was 138. ABPI = 116/138 = 0.84

Limitations:
ABPI can overestimate flow if the vessels are calcified and hardened. It is also operator dependent and will vary slightly with patient positioning. It should not be used on patients with a current deep vein thrombosis, as it risks embolisation.

ABPI Result	Interpretation	Clinical Findings
<0.5	Severe arterial Disease	Arterial ulcers, rest pain
0.5 - 0.8	Moderate arterial disease	Short distance claudication Not for compression bandaging below this point
0.8 - 0.9	Mild arterial disease	Intermittent claudication
1.0 - 1.2	Normal	
> 1.2	Calcified, non-compressible vessels, associated with diabetes Can occur at any severity of peripheral vascular disease	Correlate findings with clinical examination Compression bandaging suitable

Table 3. ABPI interpretation

Section 3: Peripheral arterial disease (PAD)

Peripheral arterial disease is a common condition typically affecting patients with other risk factors for cardiovascular disease, namely, smoking, male sex, increasing age, hypercholesterolaemia, hypertension, obesity and diabetes mellitus. Patients develop atherosclerosis and peripherally this is usually confined to the lower limbs, resulting in a reduction of arterial blood flow. They may present with either acute or chronic symptoms such as ischaemic type pain or ulcers. Typically, the initial symptoms are that of intermittent claudication. Therefore, it is important to understand the natural history of peripheral vascular disease as it can affect the management.

Intermittent claudication (IC):
This is an ischaemic type pain which usually begins after 5-10 minutes of exertion. Pain is described as an ache, cramp or numbness typically occurring in the calf but can be present in the feet or quadriceps. The pain is alleviated by rest. Another symptom is hanging their feet over the side of the bed at night to improve blood flow with gravity. At this stage trivial cuts or traumas will take longer than normal to heal. IC can be further sub-categorised into short distance claudication, where symptoms occur in less than 1 minute of exertion. It is worth noting that it takes time for the ischaemic effect to build. If patients have no pain at rest and claim to have pain after 5-10 steps, then the cause is unlikely to be vascular.

Critical limb ischaemia (CLI):
As atherosclerosis progresses, the reduction in blood flow may lead to a persistent ischaemic state. At this stage patients develop **rest pain** or pain on exertion. Patients may develop arterial, non-healing ulcers (see section 5). They may also present with gangrenous toes. It is essential that you ascertain the chronicity of any necrotic changes. CLI can either develop as a progression of atherosclerotic disease, or as an acute event (see section 3). Patients often display characteristic signs commonly referred to as the 6 P's:

- Pain
- Pallor (pale skin)
- Pulselessness
- Perishingly cold
- Paraesthesia (numbness)
- Paralysis

Acute limb ischaemia (ALI):

This is CLI caused by an acute event such as thrombosis, embolism or dissection. The common form of embolism is that of atrial thrombus, secondary to atrial fibrillation. Therefore, these patients may not have PAD.

Patients with critical limb ischaemia usually require urgent medical intervention. They must be assessed for their overall medical condition as this will affect what management options, if any, are available to them.

History and examination:
Take a history and perform a vascular examination (see Section 2). Check pulses and try to establish the likely level of occlusion. Perform Buerger's test.

Investigations:

- Check the blood tests: FBC, U&E, CRP, Clotting screen, ABG. Ensure a group and save has been taken.
- Creatinine kinase may be taken but will not provide information as to the severity of ischaemia. This should be done clinically.

General Management
Patients with intermittent claudication typically do not need urgent medical intervention. Providing their disease is stable they are managed in an outpatient setting where they can be referred for diagnostic imaging. You can advise them to see their GP to commence best medical therapy, with anti-platelet therapy and a statin.

Management of limb ischaemia should be as follows:
- Initially assess and manage the acute patient in line with CCrISP guidelines
- Resuscitate as appropriate with IV fluid replacement therapy. Use a physiological crystalloid such as Hartmann's solution
- If a patient has signs of sepsis, or clinically has an infected ulcer/wound, commence antibiotics
- Review any previous imaging available to you
- **Discuss with your Registrar early** with the above information, as this will direct the next steps
- Do not start any anticoagulation until discussion with your Senior, as the patient may be taken straight to surgery.
- In most vascular units, patients in this situation will need a CT angiogram of the lower limbs.

Following this, patients with CLI are likely to follow one of these treatment paths. Depending on the history of the presenting complaint, they may not need urgent surgery. It may be appropriate for them to undergo initial treatment and planning. Patients with ALI will often need urgent surgery to restore arterial supply to a limb.

Treatment approaches

Initial treatment with unfractionated heparin/treatment dose low molecular weight heparin, with a view to subsequent revascularisation.

Surgical:

- This may either be open surgery such as an embolectomy, or endovascular. More recently, hybrid approaches are taken combining both strategies
- If patients are not medically fit, or there are no simple interventions available, then they may undergo selective thrombolysis (depending on the availability of interventional radiology)
- Amputation (rarely 1st line in acute limb ischaemia)

Medical:

- Iloprost infusions are used for patients with microvascular disease
- Conservative management/palliation

Section 4: Abdominal Aortic Aneurysm

An abdominal aortic aneurysm (AAA) is an abnormal dilatation of the aorta. This is defined as a 50% increase in diameter but for guidelines >3cm is often used. Risk factors include: hypertension, male sex, increasing age, smoking, diabetes mellitus and connective tissue disease. In the UK there is a screening programme for those aged over 65. A single ultrasound is performed to measure the aorta. Depending on the size, follow up scans at a defined interval are performed. Aneurysms are classified by their morphology and anatomy, in particular, their relation to the renal arteries. This is important as suprarenal or juxtra-renal AAAs will typically require an open type repair. This involves placing a clamp proximal to the renal arteries during their repair and has a significant impact on mortality.

The threshold for treating asymptomatic AAAs is >5.5cm. However, this is not performed as an emergency and any surgery must be carefully planned.

During an on call you may often be called regarding patients with an incidental finding of an aneurysm. If this occurs it is important to ascertain details:

History and examination points:

- Why was the scan performed in the first place?
- What is the size of the aneurysm?
- Is the patient symptomatic?
- Is the aneurysm tender?
- Are they having ischaemic or embolic events?
- Could the aneurysm be responsible for their initial presentation requiring the scan?

Management:
Often asymptomatic aneurysms between 6-7cm can be worked up urgently as an outpatient for expedited surgery. Once aneurysms measure 8-10cm, patients may be admitted for inpatient workup. It is advised that all asymptomatic aneurysms are discussed with the Registrar on call, as many hospitals have a registry of patients on aneurysm surveillance, or awaiting surgery. They will guide as to whether or not the patient should be admitted.

Ruptured Abdominal Aortic Aneurysm

A ruptured AAA is a surgical emergency. Although the prevalence of AAA has fallen in recent years, it is still an important differential and should be an initial consideration in at-risk patients. Symptoms can be vague and may mimic other more common conditions. Patients typically present with collapse, or abdominal pain. The pain is often described as tearing or pulling in nature. It can be mistaken for renal colic. Over 50% of patients will die before they reach hospital. Mortality remains high in the group that survives to surgery.

On arrival at the emergency department, all at risk patients should have a bedside ultrasound to measure the aortic diameter. Any patient with a known AAA should be suspected for rupture, until proven otherwise.

History and examination:

- Take a history and perform a vascular examination (see section 2)
- Check for signs of retroperitoneal haemorrhage – Grey-Turner's sign (flank bruising)

- Check groin pulses for strength and symmetry

Investigations:

- Check the blood tests: FBC, U&E, CRP, Clotting screen and blood gases. Ensure a group and save has been taken.
- ECG and CXR
- The gold standard imaging investigation is a CT angiogram of the aorta - from the arch to the common femoral arteries

Management:

- Perform a thorough initial assessment of an acute patient in line with CCrISP guidelines
- Resuscitate as appropriate with IV fluid replacement therapy. Use a physiological crystalloid such as Hartmann's solution
- If a rupture is proven, then resuscitate with permissive hypotension, aiming for a systolic BP around 100.

- **Discuss with your Registrar early**. The anatomy of the aneurysm combined with the patient's physiology and medical comorbidities will dictate the management. Patients will either proceed to open surgery, endovascular surgery, or conservative management/palliation.
- Discuss with anaesthetics and intensive care early.
- If the plan is to proceed with endovascular surgery then you will need to liaise with the interventional radiology department.

Aortic dissection

An aortic dissection is created after an intimal flap is raised. Risk factors include hypertension and connective tissue disease, such as Ehlers Danlos' syndrome or Marfan's syndrome. The intimal flap can either cross over and occlude the aorta, or more commonly, rupture distally resulting in a false lumen. Branches of the aorta may then be supplied by either the true or false lumen. Although it can occur at any point, the most common starting point is just distal to the left subclavian artery. The raised flap may extend all the way down to the iliac arteries.

Patients typically present with a sudden onset shearing or tearing pain in the back, between the shoulder blades. As the flap may involve the brachiocephalic or left subclavian arteries, you may find radio-radio delay, or disparate arm blood pressure readings. If the flap involves the coeliac, or superior mesenteric arteries, they may present with visceral ischaemia.

Depending on the location where the dissection flap starts, it can be divided into two main categories:

- Stanford Type A - Dissection flap starts in the ascending, or arch, of the aorta. Treatment is surgical and urgent referral to your associated cardiac surgery unit should be made.
- Stanford Type B - Dissection flap starts distally to the left subclavian artery. Treatment is usually medical with aggressive management of blood pressure.

History and examination:

- Take a history and perform a vascular examination (see section 2)
- Check groin pulses for strength and symmetry

Investigations:

- Check the blood tests: FBC, U&E, CRP, Clotting screen, blood gases. Ensure a group and save has been taken.
- ECG and CXR
- If an aortic dissection is suspected then an urgent CT angiogram of the aorta must be requested. This is often performed by the emergency department.

Management:

- Perform a thorough initial assessment of an acute patient in line with CCrISP guidelines
- Resuscitate as appropriate with IV fluid replacement therapy. Use a physiological crystalloid such as Hartmann's solution
- Ensure that any hypertension is corrected
- For type A dissections liaise with cardiac surgery and if necessary arrange an urgent transfer.
- Type B dissections may be managed with best medical therapy providing there is no visceral involvement or aneurysmal dilatation of the aorta. If there is mesenteric or renal ischaemia, the patient may then proceed to an open or endovascular repair, depending on the precise anatomy of the dissection, as an emergency.

- Determine if there is any end organ hypoperfusion
- If an uncomplicated dissection, then contact the critical care team urgently
- The patient should be managed on critical care. They require invasive blood pressure monitoring with an arterial line.
- Critical care will manage the patient with an infusion of antihypertensives, such as labetalol.

Section 5: Ulcers

Ulcers are a common initial presentation of vascular disease. An ulcer is a breakdown of the epidermis resulting in a non-healing wound. They are commonly precipitated by a trivial trauma. However, due to vascular insufficiency the wounds are resistant to healing. They are almost completely confined to the lower limb. Upper limb ulcers are rare, they are usually a result of an infective or embolic pathology. Ulcers are broadly categorised by their aetiology into: venous, arterial and neuropathic causes. However, patients may exhibit mixed signs due to dual pathologies.

When covering a vascular on-call, it is important to be able to recognise the underlying cause of the ulcer. From there you can help to decide if a patient requires admission.

Venous ulcers

This is the most common type of leg ulcer accounting for around two thirds of cases. Venous reflux results in the stasis of blood. Wounds are unable to heal as they remain moist and congested. Typically, ulcers are confined to the gaiter area, between the ankle and knee. Wounds are often medial but they may be posterior or circumferential. They have a diffuse outline and are moist. The patient may have other venous changes such as hemosiderin deposition or lipodermatosclerosis.

Mostly venous ulcers do not require acute admission to hospital. Indications for admission include secondary infection, nursing or dressing needs and poor social support. The main course of treatment is compression bandaging. A formal surgical debridement is rarely necessary. Mostly, these can be managed by cleaning and dressing in the emergency department, or on the ward, prior to discharge. If there is thick slough, a hydrogel dressing may be used.

When assessing these patients, an ABPI must be performed. This ensures there is no co-existing arterial disease which would preclude compression bandaging. If it is a new presentation, patients must be followed up with a venous duplex scan to check for superficial reflux. From there they may be offered treatment.

Arterial Ulcers

Arterial ulcers are often the presenting sign of significant underlying arterial disease. Ulcers are commonly precipitated by a trivial trauma and are slow to heal due to poor delivery of blood. Classically, ulcers have a 'punched out' appearance and are painful. They are often found on the dorsum of the foot, or at the ankle.

Indications for admission include secondary infection, critical limb ischaemia, new necrosis of toe and large ulcers. Small ulcers may be managed with urgent outpatient investigation. If a patient is not known to have arterial disease, then the first line of investigation should be either a CT or MR angiogram, depending on local protocols. If a patient is known to have peripheral vascular disease, then an arterial duplex scan may be sufficient.

Initial treatment involves resolving any underlying infection. Wound swabs must be taken and antibiotic therapy started. Surgical treatment involves improving the blood supply to the limb with either endovascular or bypass surgery. In some cases, the flow may be sufficient to allow the wound to heal slowly without intervention.

When assessing the patient, be sure to perform an ABPI to assess for arterial disease. If there is necrotic tissue, or slough within the wound, then this must be debrided. Mostly this can be done on the ward by way of sharp debridement with a scalpel. Hydrogel or larval dressings can be used.

Neuropathic ulcers

These ulcers form over pressure areas. They are usually a result of underlying peripheral neuropathy. Specific treatment for these involves treating any underlying infection and debriding slough. From there it is important to prevent propagation of the ulcer by offloading any pressure areas. Common sites for neuropathic ulcers are the malleoli, dorsum and lateral foot.

Necrotic Toes

As with arterial ulcers, toe necrosis is often a sign of underlying arterial disease. This may either be macro, or microvascular. The digital arteries are end arteries, there is no collateral supply. Therefore, microvascular disease secondary to diabetes mellitus, may present with toe ischaemia. In this instance the foot pulses may be preserved. Patients with toe necrosis may also have underlying osteomyelitis more proximally.

Toe necrosis is gangrene. This can be classified as dry or wet:

- In dry gangrene there is progressive mummification of the digit in the absence of infection. Over time the level of perfusion will demarcate and eventually the toe will autoamputate.
- Wet gangrene is seen with superadded infection. Wet ulcers and fluid under the epidermis is seen. Often there is malodour. A toe with wet gangrene must be amputated as an emergency with the aim of preserving the rest of the foot.

It is important to distinguish whether you think the underlying cause is macro or microvascular. This can be established by taking a detailed history, performing a full vascular examination, checking the peripheral pulses and performing an ABPI. Perform an X-ray to check for osteomyelitis.

Patients with a new presentation of toe necrosis must be admitted for inpatient investigation. Initially, either a CT or MR angiogram should be performed in line with local guidance. The result of this will dictate further treatment. It is unwise to perform an amputation prior to improving the blood supply as this will result in a non-healing wound.

Diabetic foot

Patients with diabetes may present with either macro or microvascular complications secondary to their condition. Additionally, diabetes may cause peripheral neuropathy resulting in neuropathic ulcers.

Diabetes may cause progressive calcification of large vessels. In particular this occurs in the vessels below the knee. This limits blood flow and a patient may present with critical limb ischaemia. More commonly patients present with arterial ulcers or toe necrosis.

The microvascular complications of diabetes result in ulceration, or necrosis of the toes. This may result in osteomyelitis. Patients with diabetes may have preserved paedal pulses which is indicative of small vessel disease.

Patients with a Charcot joint will have additional pressure areas which may result in additional pressure ulcers. They are also more prone to develop osteomyelitis within the foot.

Ulcers:

History and examination:

- Take a history:
    - How long has the ulcer been present?
    - Ask regarding an initial traumatic event
    - Is the patient diabetic, is it well controlled?

- Perform a vascular examination, specifically:
    - Check for distribution of ulcer
    - Look for necrosis and gangrene
    - Ensure to check between the toes and under the foot

Investigations:

- Check the blood tests: FBC, U&E, CRP, Clotting screen, blood gases. Ensure a group and save has been taken.
- Perform a foot X-ray if required
- Take wound swabs

Management:

- Check for signs of sepsis. Resuscitate appropriately and treat with antibiotics in line with local protocols
- Wounds should be irrigated and dressed with a non-adherent dressing
- Determine the likely aetiology of the ulcer and order investigations appropriately

Chapter Acknowledgement

The author would like to acknowledge Mr Jamie Crinnion, Consultant Vascular Surgeon at the Royal London Hospital, for reviewing this chapter.

CHAPTER 10

MEDICAL EMERGENCIES IN SURGERY

SAMUEL MCGRATH & KEVIN O'GALLAGHER

Abstract
Section 1 – How to use this chapter
Section 2 – Assessing the acutely unwell patient
Section 3 – Key differentials for common presenting complaints

- Shortness of breath
- Chest Pain
- Delirium
- Tachycardia & ECG interpretation

Section 4 – Common medical conditions and how to manage them

- Sepsis
- Pneumonia
- Atrial Fibrillation
- Acute Coronary Syndrome
- Pulmonary embolism
- Pulmonary Oedema
- Hyperkalaemia
- Elevated blood sugars

Abstract

Whilst being on-call for surgery, you may encounter numerous medical problems with your patients on the ward. The ability to manage these problems is vital to providing effective care whilst on– call. Although undergraduate training covers medical emergencies are covered in detail, there are some specific complications and conditions that are more commonly seen in surgical patients.

Section 1: How to use this chapter?

First objective

The first objective of this chapter will be to provide a system to approach any acutely unwell patient regardless of their parent speciality. This will be using the approach: airway, breathing, circulation, disability, exposure (ABCDE). This approach should be familiar to you from Life Support Courses, such as those provided by the Resuscitation Council UK (Soar et al. 2015). We will talk through the different things to consider for each assessment.

Second objective

The second objective of this chapter is to provide an overview of investigating and managing common post-operative complications, as well as key medical emergencies.

The management of surgical patients in the post-operative period is becoming increasingly challenging as we are faced with an older, co-morbid patient population. Frailer patients are at an increased risk of developing complications after surgery, and thus, surgical on-call doctors are faced with managing problems that would traditionally present on a medical take (Roche et al. 2005, 1374) (Seymour et al. 1989, 801) (Dasgupta el al. 2009, 78).

It is important to realise that surgical patients are at an increased risk of venous thromboembolism, infection and dehydration. With this in mind, it is important to think what are the most likely differentials **for the surgical patient.** We will cover the management of the most likely differentials **for surgical patients** for common medical presenting complaints. For example, when approached with a patient with chest pain, differentials such as myocardial infarction or pulmonary embolism should be at the forefront, compared to conditions such as aortic dissection. However, it is equally important to realise that this does not mean that these pathologies do not occur, they are just less likely to occur.

The medical conditions that will be covered in this chapter are:

- Pneumonia
- Atelectasis
- Atrial fibrillation

We will also cover the following medical emergencies:

- Pulmonary embolism
- Acute coronary syndromes
- Acute pulmonary oedema
- Hyperkalaemia
- Diabetic ketoacidosis

The chapter will cover the key aspects of these conditions, as well as how to assess and investigate them. Treatment options will also be covered but please be aware that the specifics of treatment such as antibiotic choice will change from trust to trust, therefore, we always advocate prescribing in line with local policy.

Section 2: Assessing the acutely unwell patient

You will often be called to review sick patients who will have triggered the observation scoring systems, and you will also be covering patients whom you have not met before. In both these instances, the cause of the patient's deterioration will often not be immediately obvious.

It is therefore **key to have a systematic and thorough approach to assessing an acutely unwell patient.** This will allow you to safely assess them, stabilise them and will also help you remain calm in the situation. The most widely recognised system is simply following ABCDE as detailed below (Resus Council UK 2015).

Example: Doctor this patient is hypotensive and tachycardic.

From the end of the bed you will be able to gauge how sick the patient looks. In this situation, asking a basic question such as 'When did this start?' is excellent as will provide a lot of information. Can this patient complete full sentences? Are they drowsy? If the patient is very sick, rather than take a full history at this point, I would move to assessing and stabilising them.

Airway

- Is there any evidence of obstruction?
- Are they speaking in full sentences?
- Is there evidence of central cyanosis or stridor?

At this point:

- If the patient has any of signs airway obstruction, this is an acute life-threatening emergency and you need to manage the airway and seek immediate help from the on-call crash team.
- A common cause of airway obstruction is decreased consciousness – simple measures such as nasopharyngeal or oropharyngeal airways can be used as an adjunct.
- Attach high flow oxygen.
- If the patient is lying flat, sit them upright at 90 degrees (if the surgical condition permits).
- After any intervention, check the response to the intervention. If satisfactory, move onto B.

Breathing

- Are there signs of respiratory distress? - use of intercostal muscles? increased respiratory rate? decreased oxygen saturations?
- Is there tracheal deviation? (the trachea will be deviated to the opposite side in a tension pneumothorax)
- Percuss: Is there hyper-resonance? (suggests pneumothorax) Is there a dull percussion note? (Fluid or consolidation)
- Auscultate: Is there crepitation's/bronchial breathing? Unilateral or bilateral? Can you hear upper airway secretions from the end of the bed?

At this point:

- If the patient has signs of a tension pneumothorax (hyper-resonant percussion notes with absent breath sounds, tracheal deviation to opposite side) – the patient needs immediate decompression with a large bore cannula (2nd intercostal space, mid clavicular line) as per the Resus Council UK ALS guidelines (Soar et al. 2015).
- If the patient is hypoxic put them on high flow oxygen:
    - The one caveat to this is if they have a history of COPD and they are a C02 retainer. It is unlikely that you will know this information immediately, in this instance, if there is a history of COPD, start them on oxygen, complete your assessment and then review the medical notes to see if there is a history of previous C02 retention. In this subgroup, the target saturations are 88-92% and can be given controlled oxygen therapy via a venture mask, if they have COPD with no history of C02 retention target saturations at >94%.
- Arterial blood gas: perform this and ask another member of the team to run it for you. You are looking to see if the patient has evidence of respiratory failure, but it will also provide other vital information such as acid-base balance, lactate and electrolyte levels. If the patient has COPD you are looking for a raised C02. If they have a normal pH + elevated bicarbonate this may indicate chronic compensation so would be an indicator for controlled oxygen therapy.
- Move onto C

Circulation – the key here is fluid assessment: hypovolaemic vs hypervolaemic vs euvolaemia?

- Do they have cold peripheries? Are they mottled or cyanotic?
- Capillary refill time
- Pulse: is it regular or irregular? Weak or bounding? Tachycardic?
- Blood pressure: hypo or hypertensive?
- Is the JVP raised?
- Listen to heart sounds: Is there any evidence of a murmur?
- Is the urine output documented?
- Is there any evidence of peripheral oedema?

- Surgical patients often have drains – inspect these – is there high output? Is there any evidence of bleeding?

At this point:

- Obtain IV access (wide bore cannula and send blood tests including: full blood count (FBC), renal profile (U&E), bone profile, C-reactive protein (CRP), coagulation screen, group and save and if there are signs of sepsis send blood cultures). A blood gas at this point will also give important information (including acid base balance, electrolytes, Hb, lactate and blood sugar level).
- If the patient is hypovolaemic on assessment - give a fluid bolus of crystalloid. In a young fit patient, 500mls can be given stat and then assess the patient's response, in an elderly patient start with 250mls.
- Ask for an ECG – are there ischaemic changes? Is the rhythm regular?
- Move onto D

Disability– assessing the conscious level

- Calculate Glasgow Coma Score (GCS) or AVPU (alert, voice, pain, unresponsive).
- Check blood sugar
- Assess pupillary response: are the pupils equal and reactive?
- Check temperature
- Check drug chart: have any drugs been given that could cause decreased consciousness? **High doses of opiates for pain relief post operation could cause a decreased conscious level.**

At this point:

- If the GCS is less than 8, the patient cannot protect their own airway – escalate immediately
- If the BM is less than 3.5 – treat hypoglycaemia – **100mls 20% dextrose stat then reassess the blood sugar in 15 minutes** (NICE Excellence, 2019)
- If you suspect a drug-induced cause of decreased conscious level – administer the drug antagonist, for example, naloxone in opiate toxicity
- Move onto E

Exposure / Examination – particularly pertinent in a surgical patient

- Exposure the patient – look for evidence of bleeding
- Examine surgical sites
- Look for any rashes

At this point:

- **Reassess, reassess, reassess!** Reassessing the response to an intervention is a continuous process, for example, if you have administered a fluid bolus, reassess to see the response of the patient, and then decide if further fluids/boluses are appropriate.
- If the patient has stabilised proceed to take a history
- Review observation charts
- Review outstanding investigations: ECG, bloods tests
- Consider further investigations: chest radiograph, abdominal imaging.

Following this process will allow you to gather information whilst providing initial treatment to stabilise the patient. At the end of this you should have a grasp of the underlying pathology causing the clinical picture and can initiate treatment.

Section 3: Key differentials for common presenting complaints

During your assessment of an acutely unwell patient it important to draw up a list of differential diagnoses in your mind. This will help guide subsequent investigations and treatment. This is also important if you need to escalate the patient to a senior.
It is important to realise that in the context of a patient who has had recent surgery, certain differentials should be higher on your list than the non-surgical patient. Below are common presenting complaints and differentials to consider, the italic text is associated symptoms to each condition, and those in red are uncommon but must be excluded.

Please note that often an elderly patient won't simply fit into one of the categories, and if the nursing staff think there is something 'off' with the patient then this may be a sign there is an underlying problem.

Shortness of breath

- Atelectasis post surgery
  - *Pain on deep breaths, pain on coughing, fevers*
- Pneumonia (Hospital-acquired if in hospital for over 48 hours)
  - *Productive cough, fevers*
- Infective exacerbation of COPD or Asthma (important to consider if the patient has one of these conditions)
  - *Wheezy, chest feels tight, productive cough, fevers*
- Pulmonary Embolism
  - *Sudden onset breathlessness/sharp pleuritic chest pain*
  - *Remember that PE can present with haemodynamic collapse and/or cardiac arrest without any other prior signs*
- Sepsis (breathlessness due to metabolic derangement)
  - *Fevers, associated symptoms dependent on source*
- Pulmonary oedema
  - *Wheezy, SOB worst lying flat, raised JVP, may have peripheral oedema*
- Acute coronary syndrome
  - Central chest pain – 'feels like a belt around the chest', radiation to jaw and arm, nauseas, sweaty
- Pneumothorax
  - *Sudden onset breathlessness/sharp pleuritic chest pain,*
- Post surgical bleed (likelihood is dependent on operation)
  - *Symptoms dependent on site of surgery*

Chest Pain

- Atelectasis post surgery
  - *Pain on deep breaths, pain on coughing, fevers*
- Pulmonary Embolism
  - *Sudden onset breathlessness/sharp pleuritic chest pain,*
- Acute coronary syndrome
  - *Central chest pain – 'feels like a belt around the chest', radiation to jaw and arm, nauseas, sweaty*
- Pneumothorax
  - *Sudden onset breathlessness/sharp pleuritic chest pain,*
- Aortic Dissection

  - *Sudden onset tearing chest pain, radiating from centre of chest through to the back, breathlessness*

Delirium

- Sepsis
  - *Fevers, and any signs of symptoms that may suggest a source. However, an obvious source of infection may not always be immediately obvious, particularly in the elderly.*
- Hypoglycaemia
  - *Shakiness, palpations, nauseas + vomiting, headaches*
- Hyperglycaemia – need to rule out DKA
  - *Polydipsia, polyuria, nausea and vomiting, abdominal pain*
- Overuse of opiates post surgery

Tachycardia

Virtually all of the other differentials can result in a patient being tachycardic.

The most common tachyarrhythmia's you will encounter on an ECG will be a sinus tachycardia or atrial fibrillation (AF) with fast ventricular response. The commonest reasons for these rhythms to occur in a surgical setting would be response to pain, dehydration or infection, however please note that virtually all of the above differentials for other conditions can result in a patient being tachycardic.

Below are different tachyarrhythmia's that may be seen on an ECG, rather than the differentials for causes of a tachycardia. You should review all ECGs in the same systematic fashion, and some of the important questions to ask yourself are:

1. Before looking at the ECG you should assess the patient to work out the heart rate, and regularity of the pulse, and to see if there is any evidence of haemodynamic compromise
2. Is it sinus rhythm? (p-waves present or not)
3. Regular *vs.* irregular rhythm
4. Narrow *vs.* broad complex QRS

- Sinus tachycardia
    - *Regular, p- waves present, narrow complex qrs*
- Atrial fibrillation with rapid ventricular response
    - *Irregular, no p-waves, narrow complex qrs, rate >100bpm*
- Atrial flutter
    - *Flutter waves 'Saw tooth appearance of p waves', atrial rate up to 300bpm, narrow complex qrs*
- AV nodal re-entrant tachycardia (AVNRT) + AV reciprocating tachycardia (AVRT)
    - *Regular, often heart rate in 160-170 bpm, p waves may be difficult to see given the rate, p waves buried in qrs complexes 'retrograde p waves'*
- Ventricular Tachycardia (VT) – peri-arrest/arrest rhythm
    - *Broad complex QRS (>120ms), regular,*
    - *If associated with haemodynamic compromise needs urgent DC cardioversion*
    - *Requires urgent escalation to medical on call team*
- Ventricular Fibrillation – a cardiac arrest rhythm
    - You will see this rhythm in a cardiac arrest.
    - *Broad complex QRS (>120ms), irregular*

Top tips for ECG interpretation

- Are there p waves? Sinus/not sinus
- Is it regular or irregular?
- What is the rate?
- Are the QRS complexes narrow or broad?
- Are the ST segments elevated or depresed?

Figure 1. *Top tips for ECG interpretation*

Section 4: Common medical conditions and how to manage them

Sepsis

'Doctor this patient is pyrexic and looks unwell'

Sepsis is one of the most common medical problems you will have to manage on the wards. The definitions and criteria used in sepsis have changed since the introduction of sepsis-3 guidance.

> Sepsis is defined as **life threatening organ dysfunction caused by dysregulated host response to infection** (Seymour et al. 2016, 762)

The key to managing a septic patient is early identification of the infection source and administration of IV antibiotics as per the **sepsis six protocol.** All of the following criteria should be carried out **within one hour** of diagnosing sepsis.

Remember **'give three and take three'** ("Clinical – Sepsis Trust" 2019)**:**

1. Give oxygen to keep sats over 94%
2. Give IV antibiotics
3. Give a fluid challenge

1. Take a lactate measurement
2. Take blood cultures
3. Take / Measure urine output

Identifying the source of infection?

Chest and urine are common sources of infection for hospital patients. The surgical history is key when considering other sources. Has the patient had abdominal surgery? If so, could there be an intra-abdominal collection? Chest infections are also common in these patients due to diaphragmatic splinting and atelectasis. Is there any evidence of soft tissue infection at the surgical site? Skin and abdominal sources are always important to consider in surgical patients.

Pneumonia

'Doctor this patient is breathless'

Post-surgical patients are often immobile, have had prolonged hospital stays and may have been ventilated. This makes them prime candidates for hospital-acquired pneumonias (HAP). The definition of HAP is a **lower respiratory tract infection that is acquired after at least 48 hours of admission** and not incubating at the time of admission (Kalil et al. 2016, 61).

Key history points:

- Does the patient feel short of breath? – has this come on gradually or suddenly?
- Productive cough? – colour of sputum? Haemoptysis?
- Fevers?
- Chest pain? If so characterise the pain using **SOCRATES** (Figure 1). Is it pleuritic in nature?

1 **S**ite
2 **O**nset – sudden vs gradual
3 **C**haracter – Aching? Stabbing? Sharp?
4 **R**adiation – Does the pain radiate anywhere?
5 **A**ssociations – any other symptoms associated with the pain?
6 **T**ime course – Does the pain follow any pattern?
7 **E**xacerbating/relieving factors – do medications help? Is it positional?
8 **S**everity – How bad is the pain? Grade 1-10

Figure 2. *SOCRATES pain mnemonic*

Key differentials:

- Pulmonary embolism (PE) – a blood clot in the pulmonary circulation. This typically presents with sharp pleuritic chest pain, and breathlessness of **sudden** onset. This is a key differential in a post-op patient who is hypoxic and will be covered later in this chapter. In contrast, HAP will be a more gradual progression with evidence of consolidation of a chest x-ray.

- Atelectasis (see box two).
- Cardiac causes of breathlessness include arrhythmias, ACS and pulmonary oedema (see latter sections).

Atelectasis is partial collapse of the small airways in the lungs. Surgical patients are prone to this post operatively as prolonged bed rest, use of general anaesthesia, and pain post op resulting in poor ventilation are all risk factors. A chest x-ray may reveal a small area of lung collapse.

The mainstay of treatment for atelectasis is supportive therapies: 1) adequate pain relief to allow optimal ventilation, 2) chest physiotherapy and deep breathing exercises.

Figure 3. *Post-operative atelectasis*
(Schindler 2005, 341)

Key examination points:

- Signs of sepsis: pyrexia, change in mental state, hypotension, elevated respiratory rate.
- Hypoxia
- Dull percussion notes, bronchial breathing or crepitation's on auscultation, possible pleural rub

Investigations:

- Chest radiograph
- Bloods – FBC, U&E, CRP
- Blood cultures
- ABG if sats <92%

Management:

- Correct hypoxia with oxygen therapy
- Treat underlying hypotension + shock (inadequate organ perfusion)

- Antibiotics as per local guidelines
- Analgesia for pain
- Regular review, and increasing oxygen requirement is a sign to escalate

Atrial Fibrillation

Atrial fibrillation (AF) is the most common sustained arrhythmia and results from irregular electrical activity of the atria (Burns 2019). It is a common condition of the elderly and many surgical patients have a pre-operative diagnosis of AF. There are also many pre-disposing factors to atrial fibrillation, which meant that it is a common post-operative arrhythmia.

Reversible risk factors for AF
- Uncontrolled pain
- Electrolyte imbalance
- Missed medications
- Hypoxia, hypotension, hypovolaemia
- Sepsis

Figure 4. *Reversible risk factors for AF*

Many patients with atrial fibrillation will be asymptomatic, however there is a subsection of patients who can deteriorate rapidly. The main risk of atrial fibrillation is the risk of embolic stroke.

Key history points:

- Do you have chest pain?
- Breathlessness.
- Palpations – when did they start? Ask the patient to tap the rhythm out.
- Dizziness.
- Do they have a history of atrial fibrillation?

Differentials:
As per the previous section, differentials for a tachycardia include sinus tachycardia, atrial fibrillation, atrial flutter, SVT, VT. Remember some of

the key questions to ask when looking at an ECG are: Is it sinus? Is it regular? Is it broad or narrow complex?

Key examination points:

- Are they haemodynamically stable?
- Irregularly irregular pulse.
- Fluid status assessment.
- Full systems examination to look for underlying evidence of sepsis.

Investigations:

- 12 lead ECG (figure 5)
- Blood tests including FBC, U&E, bone profile, thyroid function tests
- Consider trans-thoracic echocardiogram in a non-acute setting

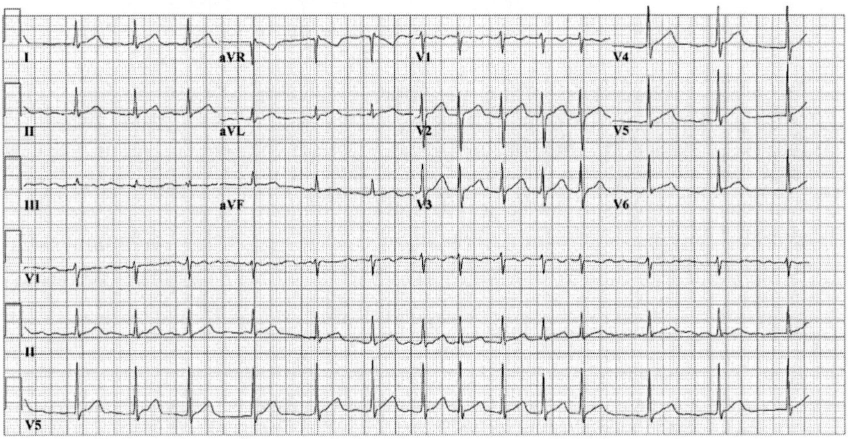

Figure 5: *ECG showing atrial fibrillation. There is no evidence of p-waves, the rhythm is irregular (the distance between each QRS complex is different). ("File:Afib Ecg (Cardionetworks Ecgpedia).Jpg - Wikimedia Commons" 2007)*

If the rate is over 100bpm, then electrical activity from the fibrillating atria is being conduced at a rapid rate, hence the term showing atrial fibrillation with a rapid ventricular response. This degree of heart rate needs to be slowed down.

Management (Kirchof et al. 2016, 2893):
This depends on the clinical situation and the chronicity of the condition. If a person has known AF then the management is different to an acute situation. Standard management strategies of atrial fibrillation are rate *vs.* rhythm control, ± anticoagulation.

For the purposes of this section we will mainly focus on acute atrial fibrillation and rate controlling AF as these are what you are likely to encounter on call. However, medical teams or the patient's general practioner should be involved to ensure this is managed correctly in the long term. This section should give surgical SHOs the confidence to identify and manage this.

Firstly:

- If the patient has haemodynamic instability, is in shock, has clear evidence of myocardial ischemia on ECG (see ACS section) or is in acute heart failure – seek senior help immediately.
- These are difficult situations where immediate synchronised DC cardioversion can is appropriate (Pitcher and Nolan 2015).

Despite the above, almost all of these patients can be managed in a ward-based setting. Many may be breathless, experiencing palpations or have mild pulmonary oedema. The key to managing these patients is to work out why the have gone into atrial fibrillation in the first place. The most common instance for this in a hospital patient is sepsis. It is important to recognise that rate control in acute AF is often difficult to achieve unless the underlying cause has been treated. (Joshi et al. 2015, 235)

Secondly:

- Look for reversible factors
    - If they have low K or Mg replace
    - Treat any underlying infection
    - Assess fluid status – are they dry post surgery? If so, give a small fluid bolus and reassess
    - Do they normally have AF and have missed their regular medicines?

- Rate control if symptomatic or rate is >100bpm
    - Beta-blockade (**contraindicated (CI) in asthma**) – 1.25mg bisoprolol and reassess, with a view to giving further beta-blockade
    - If there is a contraindication to a beta blocker, use calcium channel blocker such as diltazem
    - Consider digoxin loading (500mcg) then a repeat 500mcg/250mcg dose six hours later dependent on renal function, followed by a maintenance dose the next day. **This is a good option if there is co-existing history of heart failure.**

When to use rhythm control?
Rhythm control is the management strategy normally used in younger patients, presenting with a first presentation of symptomatic AF, with reversible precipitants corrected (this is a less common presentation in surgical patients)

Rhythm control can be electrical (synch DC cardio version) or pharmacological. If opting for electrical cardioversion then if you are outside the 48-hour hours since the onset of symptoms, or this is unclear, the patient requires 4 weeks of anti-coagulation or a trans-oesophageal ECHO prior to cardioversion (to rule out an atrial thrombus). Cases such as these should be managed by a medical team but an awareness of anti-coagulation is important for operative planning.

When to anti-coagulate?
Decisions surrounding anticoagulation for acute AF in the surgical patient can be complex, balancing the requirement for effective anticoagulation with operative considerations and bleeding risk. Out of hours, help should be sought from the senior surgical and medical team members.

Acute Coronary Syndromes

'I have chest pain'

Acute coronary syndromes (ACS) are a spectrum of conditions where the blood supply to the heart is blocked. These are split into three categories (Nickson 2016):

1. ST-elevation myocardial infarctions (STEMI) – chest pain with ST elevation or new left bundle branch block (LBBB)
2. Non-ST elevation MI (NSTEMI) - Chest pain with no evidence of ST elevation, other ischaemic ECG changes may be present such as t wave inversion or ST depression. The troponin will be raised.
3. Unstable angina – chest pain at rest, ischaemic changes on an ECG may be present but there will be no rise in troponin.

These can be fatal, particularly category one patients and have the capacity to deteriorate very quickly. A NSTEMI or unstable angina can evolve into a complete coronary occlusion (STEMI), and therefore **rapid assessment and regular monitoring of these patients is paramount**.

Key history points:

- Chest pain – patients will describe cardiac chest pain as a tight feeling, often attributed to ‘a belt being tied around the chest’
- Radiation of pain to neck or left arm
- Is the pain at rest?
- Breathlessness.
- Nausea, vomiting, sweating.
- Do they have a history of ischaemic heart disease (IHD)?
- Ask about cardiac risk factors.
- **Ask about allergies: For example, an aspirin allergy has significant implications for further treatment**

Cardiac Risk Factors

- Smoking
- Hypertension
- Diabetes
- High Cholesterol
- Family history of cardiac disease, especially at a young age
- Previous history of IHD

Figure 6. *Cardiac risk factors*

Key examination points:

- Do they look clammy, sweaty and sick?
- Are they haemodynamically stable?
- Are they desaturating?
- Do they have radial pulses bilaterally?
- Full systems examination
    - Do they have any murmurs?
    - Is there any evidence of pulmonary oedema?
    - Any abdominal pain?
    - Any pain on palpation of the chest wall?

Investigations:

- **12 lead ECG – with serial ECG's to look for dynamic changes**
- IV access + blood tests including FBC, U+E, bone profile, coagulation screen, glucose, group and save + **cardiac troponin**
- Chest x-ray

Differentials for chest pain

- Pulmonary embolism
- Musculoskeletal pain
- Pneumothorax
- Aortic Dissection
- Pericarditis

Figure 7. *Differential diagnoses for chest pain*

Management:
For the purposes of this section, we have split up the categories of ACS as their management differs. All trusts will have their own chest pain pathway to follow as individual hospitals use different antiplatelet agents, and have different troponin assays. We will talk through general management in this section, but always advocate aligning this with your local trust policy.

STEMI Management

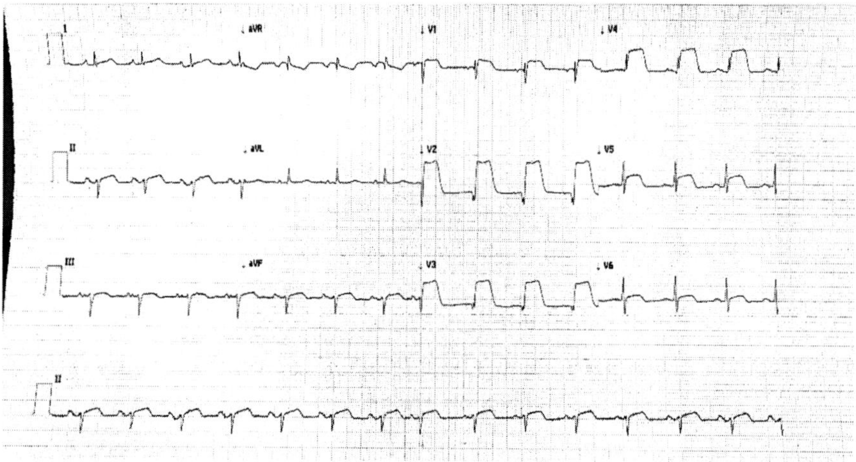

Figure 8. *ECG showing an anterior STEMI with ST elevation in V1-V6 , additionally there are q waves in V1-V3.*

In these cases, delayed treatment = increased death of heart muscle. The gold standard treatment for is percutaneous coronary intervention (PCI). If the patient meets STEMI criteria on their ECG then this requires **immediate** discussion with cardiology for transfer to a PCI centre and escalation for senior support. If primary PCI can be offered within 120 minutes of chest pain and symptoms have been present for less than 12 hours, the patient should be transferred. The immediate management is as follows (NICE 2013):

- Aspirin 300mg orally stat
- Oxygen if sats <94%
- Second antiplatelet in line with trust protocol – normally 600mg Clopidogrel or 180mg Ticagrelor
- Analgesia: 5-10mg Morphine IV + antiemetic
- Glycerine tri-nitrate GTN) sublingually – 2 puffs PRN
- Primary PCI.

STEMI Criteria: in 2 contiguous leads

Any of:

- Over 2.0mm (2 small squares) ST elevation in v2-v3 in men over 40.
- Over 2.5mm ST elevation in v2-v3 in men under 40.
- Over 1.5mm ST elevation in v2-v3 in women,
- Over 1mm ST elevation in all other leads.
- New LBBB

Figure 9. *STEMI criteria*

If the patient cannot be transferred to a primary PCI centre, careful consideration is required (by the senior team) to define alternate management. **Recent surgery is a relative contraindication to thrombolysis** therefore you registrar and consultant should be alerted immediately if a STEMI is diagnosed to facilitated quick decision making. (Ibanez et al. 2017, 119)

NSTEMI/Unstable Angina Management

On initial assessment it may not be possible to distinguish between unstable angina/NSTEMI until your troponin is back as both present with pain and ECG changes.

Initial management (NICE, 2013) (Roffi et al. 2016, 267):

- Aspirin 300mg orally stat
- Second antiplatelet in line with trust protocol
- Oxygen if sats <94%
- Morphine IV 5-10mg + antiemetic
- GTN 2 puff sublingual PRN
- Anti-thrombin therapy (Fondaparinux 2.5mg s/c in most trusts) if not contraindicated in the context of recent operation.

The next step requires risk stratification:

- Look for high risk features in presentation such as dynamic ECGs changes or worsening pain despite analgesia and initial treatment.
    - This is a high-risk MI and prompt escalation is required.

- If the patient has continual pain use IV GTN – e.g. (50mg in 50ml 0.9% saline at 1-10ml/hr, titrating to pain, and maintaining a systolic BP of over 100mmHG) and take serial ECGs
- The patient will require a repeat troponin between 3-12 hours after the initial sample dependent on the trust.
- If the troponin is elevated, this confirms the diagnosis of NSTEMI and a discussion with cardiology is warranted regarding PCI.
- Once a diagnosis of NSTEMI/UA is made, risk stratifying using scoring systems such as GRACE/HEART score will help decide on the next step in management (Grace Investigators 2001, 190).
- Early escalation of these patients is key.

Pulmonary embolism

'I feel breathless'

A pulmonary embolism (PE) is a blood clot in the pulmonary circulation, which prevents blood flow to the lungs. Recent surgery is one of the main risk factors for PE's.

Pulmonary embolism risk factors

- Deep vein thrombosis
- Immobilisation or surgery within 4 weeks
- Malignancy
- Combined contraceptive pill
- Previous VTE

Figure 10. *Pulmonary embolism risk factors*

Key history points:

- Do you feel short of breath? – was this **sudden** onset?
- Sharp, pleuritic chest pain
- PE risk factors
- Cough/Sputum production? Haemoptysis?

- The key is to rule out other causes of breathlessness such as pneumonia + ACS.

Key differentials:

- Does the picture fit with a hospital-acquired pneumonia? (fevers, productive cough, breathlessness).
- Are there any signs of fluid overload pointing towards pulmonary oedema?
- Is the chest pain typical of an acute coronary syndrome?

Key examination points:

- Hypoxia? Hypotension? Tachycardia?
- Full systems examination
    - Is the chest clear?
- Is there any calf swelling? (looking for evidence of deep vein thrombosis)
    - Is this unilateral?

Investigations:

- IV access +blood tests including FBC, U+E, CRP.
- Chest x-ray – is there any evidence of consolidation?
- 12 lead ECG – sinus tachycardia is the most common presentation of PE
- Wells score for PE (Wells et al. 2000, 416)
- ABG if hypoxic to assess if the patient is in respiratory failure.

Wells criteria for Pulmonary Embolism

1. Clinically suspected DVT — 3 points
2. PE is the number one/most likely diagnosis — 3 points
3. Tachycardia (heart rate > 100) — 1.5 points
4. Immobilization (≥ 3d)/surgery in previous four weeks — 1.5 points
5. History of DVT or PE — 1.5 points
6. Haemoptysis — 1 point
7. Malignancy (with treatment within six months) or palliative — 1 point

Interpretation

- If score > 4 and chest xray clear – CT Pulmonary Arteries (CTPA)
- If score < 4 and d-dimer blood test positive then proceed to CTPA if raised.

Figure 11. *Wells criteria for Pulmonary Embolism*

Initial management (NICE 2015) (Neff 2003,759):

- Correct hypoxia with oxygen therapy
- Analgesia for pain
- If chest x-ray shows consolidation – treat as per pneumonia section
- If the patient looks extremely sick and has haemodynamic instability or evidence of right heart strain (t wave inversion in V1-V4 or RBBB or new right axis deviation) or ischaemic changes in 2/3/avF leads: escalate immediately.
    - Treatment for a massive PE is thrombolysis. Recent surgery is a relative contra-indication to thrombolysis, therefore senior decision-making is required.
- If a pulmonary embolism is confirmed on imaging or if imaging is likely to be delayed and Wells >4, commence treatment dose low molecular weight heparin.

Pulmonary oedema

'I feel short of breath'

Patients can often receive large amounts of fluids in the post-operative period and can miss important medications peri-operatively. In somebody with a history of cardiac failure, often these small adjustments can push them into pulmonary oedema.

Key history points:

- When did the breathlessness come on? Sudden or gradual?
- Worse lying flat?
- Do they feel wheezy?
- Do they have a history of heart failure? Do they normally sleep flat?
- Do they have chest pain?
- Have they had any fevers?

Key Differentials:
If the patient is young, the diagnosis is unlikely to be pulmonary oedema secondary to cardiac failure. Other differentials for acute breathlessness include: exacerbation of asthma, pulmonary embolism and pneumonia.

Key examination points:

- Patients in acute pulmonary oedema will often be very distressed, and possibly agitated/confused secondary to hypoxia
- Haemodynamic status.
- Full systems examination:
    - Regular or irregular pulse? Is there JVP elevated?
    - Respiratory: wheeze? Is there decreased air entry or crepetations? Is it bibasal? (Left sided cardiac failure normally results in bilateral pleural effusions?
    - Heart sounds – do they have a murmur? Could this be pan systolic over the apex radiating to the axilla (mitral regurgitation) or ejection systolic parasternally (aortic stenosis).
    - Are they peripherally oedematous?
- Review fluid balance charts

Investigations:

- IV access +blood tests including FBC, U&E, CRP
- Chest x-ray – looking for blunting of the costophrenic angles (pleural effusions), patchy bibasal opacification, upper lobe diversion + fluid in the horizontal fissure.
- 12 lead ECG – is there an underlying arrhythmia? Are there any ischaemic changes? If so, send troponin (Could there be an underlying MI accounting for the deterioration)

Management (Krum and Abraham 2009) (Ponikowski et al. 2016, 891) (NICE 2014):

- Sit the patient upright at 90 degrees
- High flow oxygen
- IV furosemide 40-80mg stat – patients with poor renal function or those who are already on diuretics will require higher doses.
- Start strict fluid balance monitoring
- In hypertensive, overloaded patients' nitrate are a useful second line agent. (This is contraindicated in severe aortic stenosis)
    - 2 puffs GTN spray
    - IV GTN infusion (50mg in 50mls, normally 1-10mls/hr) – systolic BP needs to remain over 100mmHG.
- After the above, respiratory support in the form of CPAP can be considered as an adjunct treatment.
- These patients can deteriorate rapidly so always **escalate early.** An overloaded patient with persistent hypotension may require admission to HDU/CCU for inotropic support.

Signs for immediate escalation

- Signs of hypoperfusion
- Persistent hypoxia despite supplemental oxygen
- Persistent tachypnoea over 25 with use of accessory muscles
- Persistent hypotension SBP<90mmHg
- Heart rate <40 or >130 persistently

Figure 12. *Signs for immediate escalation*

Hyperkalaemia

'I am having palpations'

Severe hyperkalaemia (K>6.5mmol/L) is a medical emergency due to the risk of ventricular arrhythmias and cardiac arrest (Mushiyakh et al. 2012). Hyperkalaemia is a common problem in patients with chronic kidney disease (CKD) as the kidneys lose their ability to maintain potassium homeostasis (Kovesdy 2014, 653). It is a common problem to encounter whilst on-call and you may be contacted from the laboratory about incidental findings.

There are several mechanisms that can exacerbate hyperkalaemia in CKD, and many of these are plausible in the context of recent surgery. Examples include:

- Acute on chronic kidney injury
    - Pre-renal: dehydration.
    - Tubulo-interstitial damage – has the patient been taking NSAIDS for pain relief?
    - Post operative urinary retention causing an obstructive nephropathy
- Receiving blood transfusions (high potassium load)
- Tissue injury resulting in potassium release.
- Drug induced hyperkalaemia (K sparing diuretics, antibiotics (trimethoprim)
- Metabolic acidosis in CKD.
- Burns injuries.

Key history points:

- Be aware: hyperkalaemia can give **nonspecific symptoms**
- Nausea + vomiting
- Palpations
- Chest pain
- Generalised weakness
- Have they passed urine?

Key examination points:

- Feel the pulse? Is it regular? Are they tachycardic?
- Do they have a palpable bladder?
- Fluid balance assessment

Investigations:

- 12 lead ECG (figure 13 + 14)

ECG changes in hyperkalaemia

- Flattened p waves
- Broad QRS complexes
- Tall tented t waves

Figure 13. *ECG changes in hyperkalaemia*

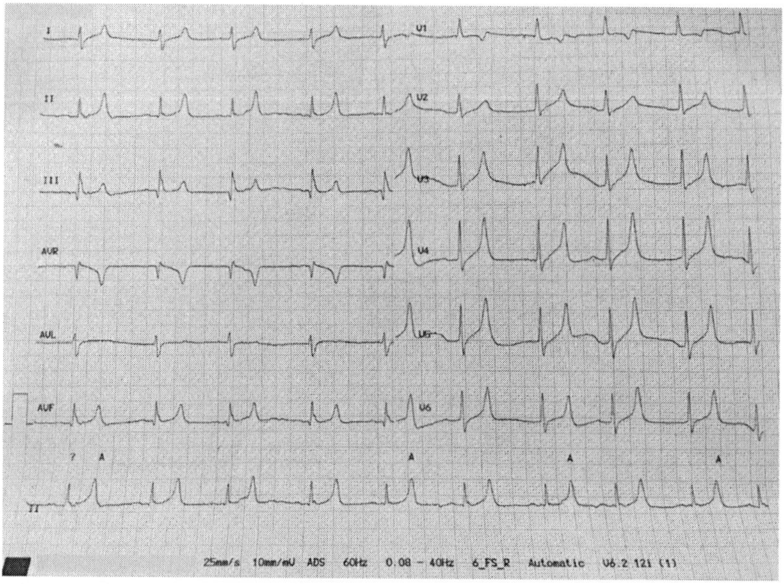

Figure 14. *ECG showing tall tented t waves in v3 –v6, leads II & III classical of hyperkalaemia (Agbayani and Gonzales 2016)*

If the patient is completely well, has normal observations and no symptoms, the sample may be artefactual. **Haemolysed blood samples can produce artificially high results.** In this instance, repeat the serum laboratory sample and also perform a venous blood gas to ensure the patient K+ is in a safe range.

Management (Maxwell et al. 2013): *Please note the majority of hospitals have a hyperkalaemia protocol to follow and treatment thresholds will differ.*

- If serum potassium is over 6.5 mmol/L, or over 6.0 mmol/L with ECG changes: treat as an emergency
    - Cardiac monitoring
    - 10ml Calcium Gluconate 10 % IV (for cardio-protection)
    - 10 units rapid acting insulin with 50mls of 50% dextrose over 10 minutes
    - Nebulised salbutamol (2.5mg)
    - Monitor serum potassium and glucose
- **If the patient has end stage renal failure and is on haemodialysis – they will require emergency dialysis and discussion with the renal team.**
- Treat underlying cause

Elevated blood sugars

'I feel sick, I feel thirsty, I feel nauseas'

Patients with diabetes can often suffer complications in the peri/post-operative period. This is a consequence of having their normal insulin regimes altered and often having a reduced oral intake. When approached with a sick diabetic patient on the wards it is important to consider the possibility of diabetic ketoacidosis (DKA) or hyperosmolar hyperglycaemic syndrome (HHS).

Diabetic Ketoacidosis

This is life-threatening that occurs most commonly in type one diabetics, but can occur in any diabetic patient on insulin. If the body lacks insulin, glucose cannot be used as a source of energy, regardless of the serum glucose concentration. In DKA, the body uses other sources, and the breakdown products “ketones” cause acidosis. DKA is more likely to occur if you are ill or have missed normal insulin doses.

Key history points:

- Thirst
- Frequent urination
- Nausea and vomiting
- Lethargy
- Blurry vision
- Abdominal pain
- Change in smell of breath? Ketones make the breath smell like pear drops
- In extreme cases: confusion or loss of consciousness
- **Are they diabetic? What’s their normal insulin?**

Key examination points:

- Full systems examination
  - Are they maintaining their airway?
  - Is there any evidence of infection?
  - Is there breathing pattern normal? Kussmaul's breathing is deep laboured breathing that occurs in a severe metabolic acidosis.
- Fluid balance assessment

Investigations:

- Bedside blood sugar
- Check ketones
  - Blood ketones is the gold standard (Nursing staff will often have a ketone meter)
  - If a blood measurement isn’t possible check urinary ketones using a urine dip
- Venous blood gas to check pH, bicarbonate and electrolytes

Diagnosis of DKA

- Ketonaemia > 3.0mmol/L or significant ketonuria (more than 2+ on standard urine sticks)
- Blood Glucose > 11.0mmol/L or known diabetes mellitus

Figure 15. *Diagnostic criteria for DKA*

Once diagnosis confirmed:

- Blood tests: FBC, U&E, CRP
- Blood cultures
- ECG
- Cardiac monitor (risk of arrhythmias secondary to electrolyte abnormalities)
- 2 large bore cannulas (one for insulin infusion and one for fluids)
- Chest radiograph if clinically indicated

Management (Dhatariya and Savage 2013):

These patients are sick, and are at a high risk of complications, such a severe electrolyte deficiencies (hypokalaemia) sepsis, acute respiratory distress syndrome and acute myocardial infarctions. They require close monitoring and the medical team should be followed immediately. All hospitals should have a DKA protocol that you can follow.

Factors requiring immediate escalation for HDU setting

- Blood ketones over 6mmol/L
- Bicarbonate level below 5mmol/L
- Venous/arterial pH below 7.0
- Hypokalaemia on admission (under 3.5mmol/L)
- GCS less than 12 or abnormal AVPU scale
- Oxygen saturation below 92% on air (assuming normal baseline respiratory function)
- Systolic BP below 90mmHg
- Pulse over 100 or below 60bpm

Figure 16. *Factors require immediate escalation for HDU in DKA*

The most important treatment is to correct the patient's fluid deficit, and then commence them on an insulin infusion. These patients are extremely dehydrated and will require large fluid volumes.

- Fluids: A 70kg adult typically will require up to 7L of fluids (100ml/kg). Sodium chloride +/- potassium is the fluid of choice. Typically give the first bag over 1hr, then second and third over 2hrs, followed by four hourly. If the serum potassium is between 3.5-5.5 mmol/L then 40mmol potassium chloride should be added to the bag. The majority of fluid given will contain potassium. If the serum potassium is less than 3.5 the patient needs to be immediately escalated.
- Commence fixed rate insulin infusion (50 units actarapid in 50mls of 0.9% saline) – commence at 0.1 unit/kg/hr. For example, 7 units per hour for a 70kg patient.
- Regular re-assessment
    - Blood ketones should fall by at least 0.5 mmol/l/hr. Alternative measurement is an increase in bicarbonate by 3 mmol/l/hr.
    - If the above does not happen then the insulin infusion will need to be increased.
    - Repeat VBG at 1 hr, then 2hrly after this to ensure acidosis is improving.
    - If glucose falls below 14 mmol/L , commence additional IV glucose 10% at 125mls per hour alongside normal saline.
    - Assess for complications of treatment such as fluid overload.

Why is potassium so important?

Serum potassium may be high on first testing but the total body potassium is low. With an insulin infusion, the potassium concentration will decrease further and can result in life threatening arrhythmias.

Figure 17. *The importance of potassium in DKA*

What if the patient isn't acidotic or ketotic?

If the blood sugar is significantly elevated (+30mmol/L), and the presentation is similar they may have Hyperosmolar Hyperglyaemic syndrome (HHS). This is a life-threatening and requires immediate escalation (English and Williams 2004, 253) (Hamblin et al. 1989, 439). The patient is in a state of extreme volume depletion and will require up to 100-200mls/kg of water for rehydration.

Diagnosis of HHS

- Hypovolaemia
- Blood Glucose > 30mmol/L with ketosis or acidosis
- Serum osmolality > 320mosmol/kg (To calculate, combine (2 (Na) + K + glucose)

Figure 18. *Diagnosis of HHS*

The mainstay of treatment is:

- Fluids: aiming to achieve a positive balance of 3-6L within the first 12 hours. 0.9% saline +/- potassium can be used as per the DKA section (Scott and Claydon. 2019).
- Blood sugar will often fall with fluid alone, and we are aiming for a decease of no more than 5mmol/L/hour. Once the blood sugar is no longer falling with fluid resuscitation, commence a low dose fixed rate insulin infusion at 0.05 units/kg/hr.
- Prophylactic low molecular weight heparin, as these patients are at a risk of venous thromboembolism.
- Regular assessment and monitoring

References

Agbayani, Michael-Joseph, and Eddieson Gonzales. 2016. "File:Hyperkalemia ECG.Jpg - Wikimedia Commons". *Commons.Wikimedia.Org*. https://commons.wikimedia.org/wiki/File:Hyperkalemia_ECG.jpg.

Burns, Dr. 2019. "Atrial Fibrillation • LITFL Medical Blog • ECG Library Diagnosis". *Life In The Fast Lane • LITFL • Medical Blog*. https://litfl.com/atrial-fibrillation-ecg-library/.

"Clinical - Sepsis Trust". 2019. *Sepsis Trust*. https://sepsistrust.org/professional-resources/clinical/.

Dasgupta, Monidipa, Darryl B. Rolfson, Paul Stolee, Michael J. Borrie, and Mark Speechley. "Frailty is associated with postoperative complications in older adults with medical problems." *Archives of gerontology and geriatrics* 48, no. 1 (2009): 78-83.

Dhatariya, Ketan, and Mark Savage. 2013. "The Management Of Diabetic Ketoacidosis In Adults". *Diabetes.Org.Uk*. https://www.diabetes.org.uk/resources-s3/2017-09/Management-of-DKA-241013.pdf.

English, P., and G. Williams. "Hyperglycaemic crises and lactic acidosis in diabetes mellitus." *Postgraduate Medical Journal*80, no. 943 (2004): 253-261.

"File:Afib Ecg (Cardionetworks Ecgpedia).Jpg - Wikimedia Commons". 2007. *Commons.Wikimedia.Org*. https://commons.wikimedia.org/wiki/File:Afib_ecg_(CardioNetworks_ECGpedia).jpg.

Grace Investigators. "Rationale and design of the GRACE (Global Registry of Acute Coronary Events) Project: a multinational registry of patient hospitalized with acute coronary syndromes." *American heart journal* 141, no. 2 (2001): 190-199

Hamblin, P. Shane, Duncan J. Topliss, Nikola Chosich, Douglas W. Lording, and Jan R. Stockigt. "Deaths associated with diabetic ketoacidosis and hyperosmolar coma, 1973–1988 (for editorial comment, see page 427; see also page 444)." *Medical Journal of Australia* 151, no. 8 (1989): 439-444.

Ibanez, Borja, Stefan James, Stefan Agewall, Manuel J. Antunes, Chiara Bucciarelli-Ducci, Héctor Bueno, Alida LP Caforio et al. "2017 ESC Guidelines for the management of acute myocardial infarction in patients presenting with ST-segment elevation: The Task Force for the management of acute myocardial infarction in patients presenting with ST-segment elevation of the European Society of Cardiology (ESC)." *European heart journal* 39, no. 2 (2017): 119-177.

Joshi, Kirti K., Mihaela Tiru, Thomas Chin, Marshal T. Fox, and Mihaela S. Stefan. "Postoperative atrial fibrillation in patients undergoing non-cardiac non-thoracic surgery: a practical approach for the hospitalist." *Hospital Practice* 43, no. 4 (2015): 235-244.

Kalil, Andre C., Mark L. Metersky, Michael Klompas, John Muscedere, Daniel A. Sweeney, Lucy B. Palmer, Lena M. Napolitano et al. "Management of adults with hospital-acquired and ventilator-associated pneumonia: 2016 clinical practice guidelines by the Infectious Diseases Society of America and the American Thoracic Society." *Clinical Infectious Diseases* 63, no. 5 (2016): e61-e111.

Kirchhof, Paulus, Stefano Benussi, Dipak Kotecha, Anders Ahlsson, Dan Atar, Barbara Casadei, Manuel Castella et al. "2016 ESC Guidelines for the management of atrial fibrillation developed in collaboration with EACTS." *European heart journal* 37, no. 38 (2016): 2893-2962.

Kovesdy, Csaba P. "Management of hyperkalaemia in chronic kidney disease." *Nature Reviews Nephrology* 10, no. 11 (2014): 653.

Krum, Henry, and William T Abraham. 2009. "Heart Failure". *The Lancet* 373 (9667): 941-955. doi:10.1016/s0140-6736(09)60236-1.

Maxwell, AP, K Linden, S O'Donnell, PK Hamilton, and GE McVeigh. 2013. "Management Of Hyperkalaemia". *The Journal Of The Royal College Of Physicians Od Edinburgh* 43 (3): 246-251. doi:10.4997/jrcpe.2013.312.

Mushiyakh, Yelena, Harsh Dangaria, Shahbaz Qavi, Noorjahan Ali, John Pannone, and David Tompkins. 2012. "Treatment And Pathogenesis Of Acute Hyperkalemia". *Journal Of Community Hospital Internal Medicine Perspectives* 1 (4): 7372. doi:10.3402/jchimp.v1i4.7372.

Neff, Matthew J. "ACEP releases clinical policy on evaluation and management of pulmonary embolism." *American family physician* 68, no. 4 (2003): 759-760.

NICE. "Myocardial Infarction With ST-Segment Elevation: Acute Management | Guidance And Guidelines | NICE". 2013. *Nice.Org.Uk*. https://www.nice.org.uk/guidance/cg167/chapter/1-Recommendations.

NICE. "Unstable Angina And NSTEMI: Early Management | Guidance And Guidelines | NICE". 2013. *Nice.Org.Uk*. https://www.nice.org.uk/guidance/cg94.

NICE. "Acute Heart Failure: Diagnosis And Management | Guidance And Guidelines | NICE". 2014. *Nice.Org.Uk*. https://www.nice.org.uk/guidance/cg187/chapter/1-recommendations#initial-pharmacological-treatment.

NICE. "Pulmonary Embolism - NICE CKS". 2015. *Cks.Nice.Org.Uk*. https://cks.nice.org.uk/pulmonary-embolism#!topicsummary.

NICE Excellence. 2019. "Hypoglycaemia | Treatment Summary | BNF Content Published By NICE". *Bnf.Nice.Org.Uk*. https://bnf.nice.org.uk/treatment-summary/hypoglycaemia.html.

Nickson, Chris. 2016. "Acute Coronary Syndromes". *Life In The Fast Lane • LITFL • Medical Blog*. https://lifeinthefastlane.com/ccc/acute-coronary-syndromes/.

Pitcher, David, and Jerry Nolan. 2015. "Peri-Arrest Arrhythmias". *Resus.Org.Uk*. https://www.resus.org.uk/resuscitation-guidelines/peri-arrest-arrhythmias/#tachycardia.

Ponikowski, Piotr, Adriaan A. Voors, Stefan D. Anker, Héctor Bueno, John GF Cleland, Andrew JS Coats, Volkmar Falk et al. "2016 ESC Guidelines for the diagnosis and treatment of acute and chronic heart failure: The Task Force for the diagnosis and treatment of acute and chronic heart failure of the European Society of Cardiology (ESC). Developed with the special contribution of the Heart Failure Association (HFA) of the ESC." *European journal of heart failure* 18, no. 8 (2016): 891-975.

Resus Council UK "ABCDE Approach" 2015. *Resus.Org.Uk*. https://www.resus.org.uk/resuscitation-guidelines/abcde-approach/.

Roffi, Marco, Carlo Patrono, Jean-Philippe Collet, Christian Mueller, Marco Valgimigli, Felicita Andreotti, Jeroen J. Bax et al. "2015 ESC Guidelines for the management of acute coronary syndromes in patients presenting without persistent ST-segment elevation: Task Force for the Management of Acute Coronary Syndromes in Patients Presenting without Persistent ST-Segment Elevation of the European Society of Cardiology (ESC)." *European heart journal* 37, no. 3 (2016): 267-315.

Roche, J. J. W., Russell T. Wenn, Opinder Sahota, and Christopher G. Moran. "Effect of comorbidities and postoperative complications on mortality after hip fracture in elderly people: prospective observational cohort study." *Bmj*331, no. 7529 (2005): 1374.

Schindler, Margrid B. "Treatment of atelectasis: where is the evidence?." *Critical Care* 9, no. 4 (2005): 341.

Scott, Adrian, and Anne Claydon. 2019. "The Management Of The Hyperosmolar Hyperglycaemic State (HHS) In Adults With Diabetes". *Diabetologists-Abcd.Org.Uk*. http://www.diabetologists-abcd.org.uk/JBDS/JBDS_IP_HHS_Adults.pdf.

Seymour, D. G., and F. G. Vaz. "A prospective study of elderly general surgical patients: II. Post-operative complications." *Age and ageing* 18, no. 5 (1989): 316-326.

Seymour, Christopher W., Vincent X. Liu, Theodore J. Iwashyna, Frank M. Brunkhorst, Thomas D. Rea, André Scherag, Gordon Rubenfeld et al. "Assessment of clinical criteria for sepsis: for the Third International Consensus Definitions for Sepsis and Septic Shock (Sepsis-3)." *Jama*315, no. 8 (2016): 762-774.

Soar, J., Deakin, C., Lockley, A., Nolan, J. and Perkins, G. (2015). *Adult advanced life support*. [online] Resus.org.uk. Available at: https://www.resus.org.uk/resuscitation-guidelines/adult-advanced-life-support/ [Accessed 26 Jan. 2019].

Wells, Philip S., David R. Anderson, Marc Rodger, Jeffrey S. Ginsberg, Clive Kearon, Michael Gent, Alexander GG Turpie et al. "Derivation of a simple clinical model to categorize patients probability of pulmonary embolism: increasing the models utility with the SimpliRED D-dimer." *Thrombosis and haemostasis* 83, no. 03 (2000): 416-42

CHAPTER 11

HELPFUL WEBSITES AND MOBILE APPLICATIONS

HUGO BEAUMONT & ROBERT MILLER

Introduction

Over recent years there have been an increasing number of available websites and mobile phone applications developed in medical and surgical fields. Although some caution is needed when using these, they can provide excellent, easy-to-use, resources when on-call.

In this chapter we will suggest helpful websites and applications with a brief description of each. There are of course many more apps, e-books, and resources available online that are not covered here. This is a selection that the authors have found helpful, particularly for on-call work. Most of these are free, however some require subscriptions for full access and some require a log-in via an institute, NHS trust, or hospital.

Disclaimer: The authors have no financial or other interest in any of the websites or apps highlighted below.

Resources relevant to all specialties: 1 → 17
Resources relevant to orthopaedics: 18 → 22
Resources relevant to plastic surgery: 20 → 26
Resources relevant to OMFS: 27 and 28
Recourses relevant to ENT: 28, 29 and 30

---

1. **E-logbook**: www.elogbook.org and elogbook app.
   This is a must-have resource for any SHO hoping to pursue a surgical career. It is a pan-speciality website allowing you to record all surgical interventions you perform or are involved with. It is important to start recording these as soon as possible in your career.

   Whatever specialty you choose to pursue, showing your aptitude in practical skills, whether in that specialty or not is important for Core Surgical Training Interviews. The logbook is then used to provide evidence for Speciality Training interviews and forms part of your review process. There is now also an app available that can be used to record cases on the go, rather than having to log into the main website.

2. **Evernote:** Evernote app
   This is a free to use app that is not specifically for clinicians. It can be used for recording and documenting lecture notes, pictures, ideas, web pages and documents etc. Within surgery, it is useful for recording key operation steps. This will allow you to refer back to them before perform the next time.

3. **DynaMed:** www.dynamed.com and DynaMed app
   This is a clinical reference tool that gathers evidence and provides objective analysis for a huge range of conditions. It provides a quick and easy-to-use tool giving an update of evidence for managing medical and surgical conditions.

4. **Up-To-Date:** www.uptodate.com and UpToDate app
   This is similar to Dynamed, providing a clinical reference tool to readily access evidence. This is not a free resource, but access is often provided via NHS trusts.

5. **E-learning for healthcare:** www.portal.e-lfh.org.uk
   This website provides helpful e-learning modules across surgical (and medical) specialties. Access is normally available via your trust, or an Athens account.

6. **ClinicalKey:** www.clinicalkey.com and ClinicalKey App
   ClinicalKey is a clinical search engine available from Elseveir. It has a wide range or resources including textbooks. It can be very helpful for accessing surgical texts in preparation for a procedure pre-operatively.

Access can be obtained through some trusts, Athens and the Royal College of Surgeons of England.

7. **Messly:** https://messly.co.uk and Messly App
This platform provides up-to-date reviews, information, and tips on training programmes, hospitals, and departments from the medical community. Furthermore, the digital tool allows you to search for locum or permanent positions to apply for.

8. **Induction:** Induction App
This is a free app giving you access to the most relevant hospital contact numbers, bleeps/pagers and door codes for the hospital you are working in. You can select your hospital and have all the contact numbers you need, instantly saving being on hold to switchboard time and time again. Furthermore, you can contribute to your hospital by adding and updating numbers on the system.

9. **Medshr:** https://en.medshr.net or Medshr App
MedShr is a free, easy, and safe way for medical professionals to discuss clinical cases and medical images. With a worldwide network of healthcare providers, it allows members to share and learn from interesting cases from around the world.

10. **Microguide:** http://www.microguide.eu or Microguide App | **RXguidelines:** http://rx-guidelines.com or RXguidelines App
These resources are a must-have for any junior doctor. They provide easy-to-use access to trust or hospital guidelines, including microbiology guidelines. Rather than having to search the trust intranet you can have the answers in a matter of seconds through these apps, making on-call decision making much more efficient and effective.

11. **British National Formulary:** https://www.bnf.org or BNF APP
This is the cornerstone of prescribing in the UK. The BNF App is invaluable. It is easy to use and can answer all your prescribing questions in minutes without having to locate a search a hard copy BNF.

12. **TouchSurgery:** https://www.touchsurgery.com or Touchsurgery App
"The Touch Surgery platform is an interactive surgical simulator for healthcare professionals; providing a realistic and detailed guide to

every step of a procedure. Users can quickly learn surgery, instantly test their knowledge, and rehearse for surgery." - Touchsurgery.

Touchsurgery allows you to view the key steps of operations prior to performing or observing them. This allows for an interactive resource to help learn and prepare how to perform operations in a safe environment.

13. **MDCalc:** MDCalc App
    This is a free and comprehensive tool for medical professionals, making it easy to perform medical calculations, calculate scores, scales and classify pathologies (e.g. GCS and Wells DVT score), improving your documentation, handover, and management of patients.

14. **Radiopaedia:** www.radiopaedia.org
    This is a great website for understanding radiology images and improving your radiology knowledge with case reports and key findings.

15. **BMJ Best Practice:** https://bestpractice.bmj.com/info/ or BMJ best practice App
    This resource provides fast and easy access to the latest evidence-based information on diagnosis and treatment for healthcare professionals. You must however have a valid BMJ subscription (this is free with any BMA membership).

16. **iResus App**
    This is a free tool allowing healthcare professionals access the latest algorithms from the 2015 resuscitation council (UK) guidelines quickly and easily. This can be very helpful when on-call, either as an aide-memoir or if not familiar with some of the more complex algorithms.

17. **Siilo:** Siilo App
    Siilo is a secure messaging app for medical professionals, on which you can safely share confidential patient information, including names, hospital numbers, and identifying photos (e.g. ECGs). It's very useful when trying to get quick advice from seniors on your team while on-call. However, we would advise checking with your trust prior to using it, as often trusts have specific advice regarding the use of messaging apps and clinical information.

18. **Orthobullets:** www.orthobullets.com or orthobullets App
This is general reference guide for all things orthopaedic and includes multi-choice questions and useful pictures.

19. **Orthoconsent:** http://www.orthoconsent.com
This is a useful guide to consenting orthopaedic patients for theatre with rough percentage risks of each complication. Remember however, you should only consent patients for operations you are happy to perform yourself.

20. **BOA Standards for Trauma (BOASTs)**:
https://www.boa.ac.uk/publications/boa-standards-trauma-boasts/
These guidelines have been developed by the British Orthopaedic Association and provide guidelines on the best practice management for a range of fractures, orthopaedic, and trauma conditions.

21. **Wheeless' Textbook of Orthopaedics:**
http://www.wheelessonline.com
This is a free online textbook coving the entire orthopaedic specialty – what more could you ask for?

22. **AO Surgery Reference**: www2.aofoundation.org/wps/portal/surgery or AO Surgery Reference App.
This is a great resource to help guide the management of fractures, including fixation methods and guides on how to perform operations.

23. **Mersey Burns App**
This a fantastic free clinical tool for anyone working with burn injuries. It allows you to easily calculate burn area percentages and establish fluid prescribing regimes.

24. **Hand Therapy App**
This app has been developed by the hand therapy team at Chelsea and Westminster Hospital. It provides details of all hand rehabilitation programs following hand and wrist injuries and operations. It is helpful for both patients and clinicians delivering advice regarding hand physiotherapy.

25. **Wikiplastics:** www.wikiplastic.surgery, or WikiPlastic App
Wikiplastics is a peer learning plastic surgery video sharing platform, on which you can view or upload videos of up-to-date surgical techniques and lectures related to plastic surgery.

26. **HIPE App**
The guidelines within this app have been developed, written and published by the Oxford University Hospitals Plastic Surgery Department. Although the guidance on who to contact and how is specific to the Oxford University Hospitals, it provides an easy to use decision aid when assessing plastic surgery referrals in ED. Use the guidelines to discuss cases with referrers over the phone or before you see a patient to give an idea of the correct and safest pathway. They will also provide a reminder for the actions that ED /referring units are required to take.

27. **Dental trauma guide online:** https://dentaltraumaguide.org
The Dental Trauma Guide is a web-based tool for evidence-based dental traumatology. To get access to the full Dental Trauma Guide you need to become a certified DTG member (as of January 2017).

28. **National Tracheostomy Project**: http://www.tracheostomy.org.uk and NTSP App
This provides Emergency Tracheostomy and Laryngectomy algorithms both online and on an app. There are also helpful video moulages taking you through emergency scenarios.

29. **ENT SHO:** ENTSHO.com or ENTSHO App
This is a really useful guide that can be used as an app on your phone whilst on-call providing accessible ENT advice for doctors and nurses. It is especially targeted at junior doctors covering ENT and professionals in emergency and primary care.

30. **ENT UK Patient information leaflets**:
https://www.entuk.org/patient-information-leaflets-1
These are convenient patient information leaflets - ideal for explaining conditions, or can be used to guide patients to information.

EDITOR BIOGRAPHY

Mr Robert Miller is a plastic surgery registrar currently working at the Royal London Hospital, London, UK. After graduation from the University of Bristol with a first-class Degree in Neuroscience and an MBChB he completed his foundation training in Oxford, progressing to surgical training in London. Over this time, he has covered at least eight surgical specialties whilst on-call, with varying levels of experience in each. This, together with an interest in surgical training and education, provided the motivation for developing this book in order to support fellow surgical juniors provide high-quality and safe care (with minimal stress!) whist on-call. Although still in the early stages of a surgical career, Robert has over 25 publications in peer-reviewed journals, has presented work at national and international meetings, won national prizes in surgery, authored book chapters and taught/tutored/examined at Oxford University, University College London and Barts and The London School of Medicine and Dentistry. Outside of Medicine he has a strong musical background. He has a Diploma in trumpet performance, has performed in some of the country's most prestigious concert venues and he has published a book to help young players learn trumpet scales using a novel colour-based method based on the principles of implicit memory ("Smarties for Brass").

LIST OF CONTRIBUTORS

Mr Abdul Kasem; MD, Dip, MRCS, AFRCS, FRCS (Ed), FRCS (Eng) (Consultant in Oncoplastic Breast Surgery; Princess Royal University Hospital, Kings' College Hospital NHS Foundation Trust)

Mr Christos Kontovounisios; MD, PhD, FACS, FRCS (Consultant Surgeon; Department of Surgery and Cancer Chelsea & Westminster and the Royal Marsden Hospital, Clinical Senior Lecturer in Colorectal Surgery at the Department of Surgery and Cancer Imperial College)

Dr Hugo Beaumont; BSc (Hons), BMBS, (Foundation Doctor; Royal United Hospitals Bath)

Mr Iain Yardley; BM, MPH, FRCS (Consultant neonatal and paediatric surgeon; Evelina London Children's Hospital, London)

Mr Indran Balasundaram; MBBS, BDS, BSc (Hons), MRCS (Eng), FRCS OMFS (Eng) (Consultant Maxillofacial Surgeon; Imperial College NHS Trust)

Ms Jennifer Martin; MBBCh, MEd, MRCS (Registrar in Urology; South-West Deanery)

Ms Jessica Lunn; BSc, MBChB, MRCS (CT2 in Ear, Nose and Throat surgery; St George's Hospital, London)

Mr John Pascoe; BMBS, MRCS, PGCert (ClinEd) (CT2 in Urology; Musgrove Park Hospital, Taunton)

Dr Kevin O'Gallagher; MRCP, MBBS, BA(Hons) (MRC Clinical Research Fellow and Interventional Cardiology Registrar, King's College London and King's College Hospital NHS Foundation Trust)

Mr Mark Mikhail; BSc, MBBS, MRCS (Plastic Surgery Registrar; Wexham Park Hospital, London)

Mr Oliver Beaumont; BSc (Hons), MBChB, MRCS (ST3 registrar in Trauma and Orthopedics; Bristol Royal Infirmary, Bristol)

Mr Oliver Gosling; MBChB, FRCS (T&O) (Consultant Trauma and Orthopaedic Surgeon; Musgrove Park Hospital, Taunton)

Mr Raj Lakhani; BSc, MBBS, DO-NHS, MRCS, FRCS (ORL-HNS), MSc (Consultant Rhinologist, Facial Plastics & ENT Surgeon; St George's Hospital, London)

Mr Robert Miller; BSc (Hons), MBChB, MRCS (Registrar in Plastic and Reconstructive Surgery; Royal London Hospital, London)

Ms Sally Jay; BMedSci, BMBS, MMedSci (Medical Education), FRCS (Plast) (Consultant Plastic Surgeon; Oxford Radcliffe Hospitals, Oxford)

Dr Sam McGrath; BSc, MBChB, MRCP (ST3 Registrar in Cardiology; Conquest Hospital, Hastings)

Mr Simon McCluney; BSc, MBChB, PGCAP, MRCS (Registrar in Paediatric Surgery; Evelina London Children's Hospital, London | Registrar in General Surgery; Chelsea and Westminster Hospital, London)

Mr Toby Visholm; BMedSci (Hons), BMBS, BDS, MRCS (Oral and Maxillofacial Surgery Registrar, John Radcliffe Hospital, Oxford)

Mr Tom Pampiglione; BMBS, MRCS (Vascular Surgery Registrar; Royal London Hospital, London)

Mr Zachary Cole-Healy; MBCHB (Hons), BDS (Hons), BMedSci (Hons), PGCert, MRCS (ST1 Oral and Maxillofacial Surgery, North West Region)

Ms Virginia Caddick; MA (Cantab) in Natural Sciences (Biological), MBChB (Hons), MRCS (ST3 Registrar in Breast Surgery at Princess Royal University Hospital, Kings' College Hospital NHS Foundation Trust)